Recovering from Breast Surgery

Exercises to Strengthen

Your Body and

Relieve Pain

Diana Stumm, P.T.

Alameda CA

Acknowledgement is made to the National Cancer Institute for the
illustrations that appear on pages 89-90, which originally appeared in *Breast
Exams: What You Should Know*, NIH Publication No. 93-2000.

Library of Congress Cataloging-in-Publication Data
Stumm, Diana.
Recovering from breast surgery : exercises to strengthen your body and
relieve pain / Diana Stumm. — 1st ed.
p. cm.
Includes bibliographical references and index.
ISBN 0-89793-180-7
1. Breast—Cancer—Surgery. 2. Breast—Cancer—Patients—Rehabilitation.
I. Title.
RD667.5.S78 1995
616.99'449059—d:20 95-3153

Project Editor: Lisa E. Lee   Production Manager: Paul J. Frindt
Cover Design: Jil Weil Design   Book Design: Kathleen Szawiola
Illustrations: Dave Titus   Copy Editor: Colleen Paretty
Proofreaders: Susan Burckhard, Lara Thompson
Index: ALTA Indexing Service
Sales & Marketing: Corrine M. Sahli   Publicity & Promotion: Darcy Cohan
Customer Support: Sharon R.A. Olson, Sam Brewer
Order Fulfillment: A&A Quality Shipping Services
Administration & Rights: María Jesús Aguiló
Publisher: Kiran S. Rana
Set in Aldine and Egyptian by 847 Communications, Alameda CA
Printed and bound by Publishers Press, Salt Lake City, UT
Manufactured in the United States of America

9 8 7 6 5 4 3 2   First edition

Ordering Information

Trade bookstores and wholesalers in the U.S. and Canada,
please contact

Publishers Group West
1700 4th St.
Berkeley, CA 94710
Telephone 1-800-788-3123 or (510) 528-1444
Fax (510) 328-3444

Special Sales

Hunter House books are available at special discounts when
purchased in bulk for sales promotions, premiums, fundraising.
For details, please contact

Special Sales Department
Hunter House Inc.
P.O. Box 2914
Alameda, CA 94501-0914
Telephone (510) 865-5282
Fax (510) 865-4295

College textbooks/course adoption orders

Please contact Hunter House at the address and phone
number above.

Orders by individuals or organizations

Hunter House books are available through most bookstores or can
be ordered directly from the publisher by calling toll-free

1-800-266-5592

Acknowledgments

I would like to express my heartfelt appreciation to the following people, each of whom has contributed to the completion of this book.

Marilyn Woods, P.T., who started me on my way.

Phyllis Anderson, who taught me what women recovering from breast cancer need to know.

Hewlett Lee, M.D., and the late John Kieraldo, M.D., who introduced me to the great need for the role of physical therapy in the recovery from breast cancer.

To the five physicians who have faithfully supported and encouraged my work:

Francis A. Marzoni, M.D., general surgery, Palo Alto Medical Foundation;

M. Ellen Mahoney, M.D., general surgery, Palo Alto, California;

M. Richard Maser, M.D, plastic and reconstructive surgery, Palo Alto Medical Foundation;

Jane Marmor, M.D., radiation oncology, Sequoia Hospital, Redwood City;

Paula Kushlan, M.D., oncology, Palo Alto Medical Foundation.

Also to Sherry Blair, who patiently helped me "tame" the computer.

Tita McCall, who believed in me and in this book, and made sure the dream became a reality.

• • •

This book is written to honor the women who sought my help and left me with this legacy of their wisdom, which I now share with you.

Contents

Contents *(continued)*

List of Exercises

List of Exercises (continued)

Important Note

The material in this book is intended to provide a review of stretching exercises and self-care measures for breast surgery recovery. The contents of this book have been reviewed by medical experts and every effort has been made to provide accurate and dependable information. However, health-care professionals have differing opinions and there are continual advances in medical and scientific research, so some of the information may become outdated.

The publisher, author, and editors cannot be held responsible for any error, omission, or dated material. Any of the treatments described herein should only be undertaken under the guidance of a licensed health-care practitioner. The author and publisher assume no responsibility for any outcome of the use of these treatments in a program of self-care or under the care of a licensed practitioner.

If you have a question about the appropriateness of the treatments described in this book, please consult your health-care professional.

. . . .

Preface

If you are like most women who undergo treatment for breast cancer, you probably know more about the disease and the procedures used to fight it than you do about recovery. This book will change that.

Cancer is a particularly unkind disease. Usually, when you get sick you feel bad first and treatment helps you feel better. With breast cancer, you feel just fine and then you learn you have cancer. The onset is usually painless; it doesn't warn you. You start to feel bad *because* of the treatments. The women who come to me following treatment have had no time to prepare a defense or a strategy for their recovery.

The experiences you will soon read about are from those women. Their stories represent the voices of hundreds of determined and courageous women who want to tell you what they have learned about recovering from breast cancer. "Put this down on paper," they repeatedly urge me. "Help us tell the women coming behind us what we have learned."

An impressive network of inspired women are eager to increase understanding and communication about breast cancer, and to improve the quality of treatment and recovery. During the 27 years I have been working with breast cancer patients, the medical and political climate has changed dramatically. Women now have options that did not exist a few years ago. In the 1960s and early 1970s, a patient went under general anesthesia and into surgery not knowing whether she would wake up with just a biopsy scar or a missing breast. Today, a woman can actively participate in choosing the treatment that is most likely to cure her of the disease and decide whether to keep her breast.

Women, both those with the disease and not, have demanded changes in medical treatment protocols, in legislation about patient's rights, and in the insurance coverage of diagnostic and treatment procedures. Now efforts are directed at raising the funds needed to find a cure. Overall, there is no question in my mind about the contribution these women have made toward making the practice of medicine more humane. Let them help you, too.

Diana Stumm
Spring 1995

ONE

So, the Surgery Is Over—Why Am I Not Getting Better?

As I greeted Barbara in the waiting room, I could see the question in her eyes even before she spoke: "Can you help me with this pain?" I had seen this expression hundreds of times before in my career as a physical therapist specializing in the rehabilitation of breast cancer patients. Like hundreds of thousands of American women before her, Barbara had undergone surgery for breast cancer. In her case, the surgical procedure was a lumpectomy followed by an axillary dissection, or the removal of lymph nodes from under her arm. Barbara had expected the incisions to hurt; what took her by surprise was the unrelenting pain under her arm that seemed to be getting worse instead of better. Instead of being able to use her arm normally soon after surgery, as she had planned, she was in pain, deeply troubled, and wondering what she was doing wrong.

Barbara was not doing anything wrong. She just desperately needed information about what to do after her surgery. She was tense, anxious, and depressed because she did not understand how her body was reacting. Barbara had not given much thought to what she would feel like *after* the surgery; all of her energy and courage had gone into just getting *through* it.

Faced with the diagnosis of breast cancer, a woman has an overwhelming series of decisions to make—while she is in

1

shock and disbelief, and dealing with the stress of having a life-threatening disease. She may not feel she has adequate time to research her treatment choices. She may not be able to hear clearly and absorb the options described by her physicians. The choices may be both terrifying and repugnant to her, but eventually she makes one. What she may forget is to ask important questions about her life as a result of these decisions. After the surgery, what will she look like? How will she feel? How well will she be able to function? How much pain can she expect and for how long? When will her arm be normal again? Few know to ask: what can *I* do for myself, to speed my recovery and avoid unnecessary complications?

Most women who have breast surgery are not prepared for prolonged pain and loss of function. Some do have very smooth recoveries with minimal discomfort and inconvenience, and are able to resume their lives without doing specific exercises or seeking professional guidance. More women, however, experience disabling effects after surgery. Over and over again they say, "Why didn't they tell me this might happen? Why wasn't I better prepared?" Unfortunately, there is very little published information about the *physical* aftereffects of breast cancer treatments and the rehabilitation techniques that help women recover. Reading about *why* you are feeling the way you are will help you know that your reactions are not unusual.

This information is useful if you have just learned you have cancer and must decide which surgery is most appropriate for you. It can also help if you are in the middle of your treatments and are trying to restore your life to normalcy but are held back by pain or loss of function. It is even a valuable resource if you have been treated for breast cancer months or years ago but are frustrated because you are not yet back to your full physical and emotional potential. You may also discover that reading the book again a few weeks or months down the line will clarify some ideas that may have gotten muddled during the rush to make early critical decisions.

... How This Book Is Organized

This book discusses the treatments, complications, rehabilitation procedures, and stages of recovery common to breast cancer patients in the following way. Chapter 2 presents a review of the basic anatomy of the breast and adjacent lymphatic system, followed by an explanation of each surgical procedure, and the common physical sensations and limitations of movement that often result. Chapters 3 through 8 use the stories of typical women to illustrate the different problems that arise with a particular procedure or topic. While every woman's experience is unique, you will find these stories represent a range of common physical and emotional responses. Do keep in mind that there is a variety of reactions, and *all* are normal.

Each chapter discusses and is often followed by specific exercises designed to relieve the pain of surgery, strengthen muscles, and help you regain control of your body. There are basic exercises to restore shoulder motion, as well as exercises that are more specific for particular surgeries. Each is described and illustrated in detail. Most exercises, particularly those for restoring basic shoulder motion outlined in Chapter 3, are appropriate for anyone who has had breast surgery that includes axillary lymph-node dissection.

You can read this book straight through or flip to the chapter that interests you. Different exercises are presented in each chapter and several may be appropriate for you, not just those presented in the chapter you identify with the most.

You can take your recovery into your own hands by setting aside time every day to do these simple stretch, strengthening, and fitness exercises. Even if you have never done regular exercise before and resist the idea, don't feel overwhelmed. You *can* do this if you make up your mind to do it. Thousands of women of every size, shape, and lifestyle have already accomplished this. And they encourage you to join them. The sooner you get started on your program of "self-therapy," the sooner you will see results. Resolve to give it a try.

If you are already committed to a regular fitness regimen, try to be patient with yourself. You may feel as if you are back in the first grade for awhile, but I promise that the work and discipline you have already put into conditioning your body will see you through this experience faster and more smoothly than other women. This is because you have already learned to listen to your body, you have an idea of your body's capabilities, and you know the value of exercise.

••• The Referral Process

If you find you need help beyond the advice in this book, help is at hand. Physical therapy is not an automatic part of your hospital recuperation, but it may be necessary. Most women are not in the hospital long enough to have a physical therapist visit them, and most surgeons do not routinely refer you to one. If you have any question that you might need professional guidance with these exercises, ask any of your doctors (it does not have to be the surgeon) to refer you to physical therapy as an outpatient. Your hospital probably has a physical therapy department that treats both inpatients and outpatients. If not, there are therapists in clinics and private practices in most communities. Remember that it is appropriate for you to ask for professional help *any time* during the recovery process. If you cannot reach overhead or easily put your hand behind your head by three weeks after surgery, or if you are experiencing excessive pain, you need help. Payment for physical therapy can usually be taken care of by insurance, and this usually requires a doctor's referral. HMO-type health plans offered through your or your spouse's place of employment often have stricter rules requiring prior authorization from a representative of the insurance carrier. In other cases, you may have to pay for the visits up front, and the insurance company will reimburse you. Sometimes you need to pay only a co-payment for each visit, and the therapist bills the insurance company for the rest of the fee. Some companies prefer to be billed directly by the provider. Keep in mind that even if you have no insurance, a great deal can be accomplished by paying for one or two instruction sessions. More than anything else, you need to know how to proceed safely with an exercise program that is designed to restore your shoulder and arm mobility to normal levels.

• • • Healing All of You

At the time you learned you had breast cancer, you were probably feeling just fine. Suddenly you found yourself lying on examination tables, exposed and unprotected. Concerns that were monumental yesterday became trivial. As the news sank in, you felt your life go out of control. The medical tests, surgery, and other treatments that follow the diagnosis intensified that feeling of loss of control. You started to feel bad not because of the disease but because of the treatments. This book is about helping you to feel better and regain control. Its purpose is to help you learn what *you* can do for *yourself* to feel strong again. It is intended to be a guide along the road back from helplessness.

You will learn how to look at your physical *and* emotional needs in a new way. You are ready to feel strong again, to be back in control of your body and your life. Yesterday you may have been preoccupied with pressures or deadlines at your job, or with concerns about your family and friends. Now your body and your feelings are demanding your immediate attention. *You* are now your primary focus, and this is entirely appropriate. There is no "wrong way" to feel. To successfully cope, you need to develop a plan of action to deal with your feelings, and put it into practice.

This book will help you take better care of yourself. It will also help you know when your own efforts may not be enough, and when you need to seek professional guidance. Finally, remember that you are not alone. Thousands of women have been down this path to recovery before you. Expert help and support are available—and with the necessary knowledge and encouragement, you can experience what it means to heal *all* of you.

Before Therapy: A Medical and Physical Overview

There is a vast amount of information available about how breast cancer is diagnosed, the different types of tumors, and the surgical procedures for treatment; this information can be found in health books and medical journals. There are also several personal stories written by breast cancer survivors that describe the psychological impact and emotional experiences of having breast cancer. Many communities have health libraries affiliated with their hospitals, which have volunteers and computerized indexes to help you locate these publications. This chapter gives you an overview of breast anatomy and brief descriptions of common procedures, then focuses on what to expect as a result of treatment.

· · · The Breast and Lymphatic System: A Road Map

The female breast is composed of milk glands (or lobes), milk ducts, and fatty, fibrous tissue. The milk glands produce milk after the birth of a baby and the ducts transport the milk from the glands to the nipple. The breast is supported by skin and fibrous bands called Cooper's ligaments. It rests on top of the large chest muscle, the *pectoralis major*. There is

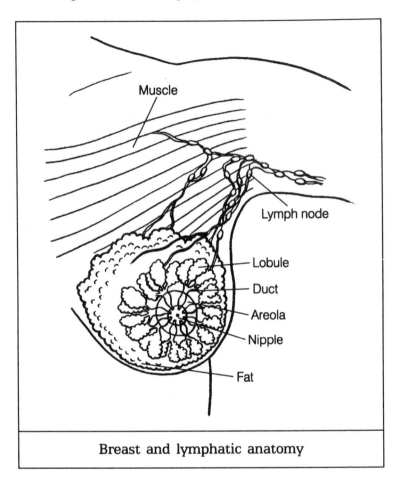

Breast and lymphatic anatomy

no muscle in the breast itself. Breast tissue tends to be more dense and fibrous in younger women, and more soft and fatty in older women.

The lymphatic system is the part of the circulatory system that drains lymph from tissue. *Lymph* is the fluid that bathes the individual cells of the body and transports the waste products of metabolism. The system is composed of narrow tubes and bean-shaped filters called lymph nodes. The tubes, or lymph vessels, transport the lymph back to the large blood vessels near the heart, where it is combined with the bloodstream. The nodes are filters that trap foreign matter, such as bacteria and cancer cells, as the lymph passes through them. Lymph nodes are found throughout the body: in the abdominal and chest cavities, in the neck, the limbs, and where the limbs join the trunk of the body. There are layers of lymph nodes along the side of the chest and under the arm that filter the lymph fluid draining from the breast and the adjacent arm. Unlike the arteries, where there is pressure resulting from the force of the heartbeat, there is no pressure pushing the fluid in the lymphatic system. Lymph moves partly as a result of osmosis, which causes fluid to flow through a membrane to equalize the concentration of fluid on both sides of the membrane. The walls of the lymph vessels are porous membranes. Lymph is pushed along the vessels by the pumping action of muscles working in the limb.

When a biopsy determines that a breast lump is cancerous, surgery is the next step, because the surgeon must remove some of the armpit or axillary lymph nodes to stage the disease. *Staging* is the medical term for examination of the lymph nodes microscopically by a pathologist to determine whether the cancer is confined to the breast or if it has spread into or beyond the lymph nodes—essential information to establish the necessity and course of later treatments. Lymph nodes will trap some of the cancer cells if they leave the breast. If cancer cells are present in the removed nodes, further treatments will be recommended. *It is the unavoidable surgical damage to the lymph vessels that pass through the lymph nodes that causes much of the pain and shoulder tightness that women feel after breast cancer surgery.* In the future, fewer axillary lymph-node dissections will be performed. As diagnostic procedures become more technologically sophisticated, it will become possible to stage cancer and recommend treatments with less surgery.

• • • Surgery

Once a biopsy has shown a breast lump to be malignant (invasive cancer), a woman has two choices of surgical treatment. One is *lumpectomy,* also known as partial mastectomy or segmental mastectomy. This means that just the part of the breast containing the tumor is removed. The other choice is *mastectomy,* which is removal of the entire breast. Regardless of which procedure she undergoes, a woman is also likely to have an *axillary lymph-node dissection.* (*Axilla* is the medical term for the armpit area.) Although each procedure requires a different incision, the impact on the lymphatic system is the same.

Lumpectomy

If the tumor is caught early enough, a woman can probably choose to have a lumpectomy. She will then undergo a three-part procedure: one, the lumpectomy, or removal of the tumor itself; two, an axillary lymph-node dissection that requires a separate three-to five-inch incision in the armpit (this may be done separately from the lumpectomy and requires general anesthesia); and three, six or eight weeks of daily radiation therapy treatments to the remaining breast tissue. The lumpectomy takes out the primary tumor of cancer cells and the axillary lymph-node dissection stages the disease. If the tumor was actually removed rather than sampled at the time of the biopsy, then the surgeon may return to the site to take out additional tissue to create good margins, that is, to be sure a "moat" of healthy cells surrounds the area where the tumor was. Radiation therapy is necessary because cancer cells can grow simultaneously in other locations in the same breast, separate from the main tumor. The radiation will destroy these cells before they can organize themselves into other tumors. A woman who chooses to save her breast is choosing to have radiation therapy.

Mastectomy

When a mastectomy is performed, the entire breast is removed while the patient is under general anesthesia. There are three types of mastectomies: simple, modified radical, and radical. By far the majority of mastectomies performed today are modified radical mastectomies. This means that the entire breast and some of the axillary lymph nodes are removed simultaneously. Only one incision is made, across the chest. Radical mastectomy requires the removal of the breast, plus all or part of two chest muscles: the pectoralis major and the pectoralis minor, and all of the lymph nodes under the arm. This type of mastectomy is rarely done now; it is done if the tumor is very large or the cancer has directly invaded the chest muscle. Modified radical mastectomy became the preferred operation when researchers discovered that the survival rate for patients was the same with a less disabling procedure.

Simple mastectomy, or removal of the breast tissue alone *without* lymph node dissection is performed when one of three circumstances applies. The first is when a woman is diagnosed with *ductal carcinoma in-situ* or noninvasive cancer. This type of cancer must still be completely removed surgically because, if given enough time, it could become invasive and spread to other parts of the body. Lymph nodes are not usually taken out for in-situ tumors that are caught early, because these tumors are contained in the walls of the ducts and do not spread into the lymphatic system. The second circumstance is when the breast is being removed prophylactically, that is, to prevent cancer from developing. Some women who have had breast cancer and have a high risk of developing cancer in their other breast choose to have that breast removed as a preventive measure. Other women may have a strong family history of breast cancer. Rather than being "next in line," they may decide to have both breasts surgically removed before the cancer has time to develop. The third situation calling for a simple mastectomy is when a woman declines to have an axillary dissection, or when her physicians believe that the decision to use chemotherapy or hormone therapy will not be affected by her lymph node status.

Axillary Lymph-Node Dissection

When a surgeon removes the fatty tissue from the armpit containing the lymph nodes, the effect on the skin resembles a tuck taken in the armpit. This is true regardless of whether the axillary dissection is performed simultaneously with a mastectomy or as a separate incision in combination with a lumpectomy. Surgeons have found that obtaining an average of 10 to 20 lymph nodes is sufficient for pathological staging and causes fewer complications than going higher into the armpit for a larger sampling (30 to 50 nodes). When the tissue under the arm containing the lymph nodes is removed and the skin is drawn back together, the concave surface of the armpit is now deeper and the skin is pulled together tighter than it was before the surgery. As it heals, the skin along the incision often puckers, causing one or more folds to form in the skin along the underside of the arm. These skin folds contain the severed lymph vessels, which dry up and draw taut, temporarily reducing shoulder mobility.

Another less common complication of axillary dissection is the temporary loss of function of one of the muscles that stabilizes the shoulder blade. This is the broad, fan-shaped muscle, the *serratus anterior,* which holds the shoulder blade against the back of the rib cage. Because the motor nerve that carries the messages from the brain to the muscle passes through the armpit, this muscle is sometimes affected. When operating, the surgeon may need to gently move the nerve to reach some of the lymph nodes. Removing tissue from around the nerve may disrupt its blood supply, causing the nerve to go into shock and shut down. Because the muscle is temporarily not receiving messages from the brain, it stops functioning, causing the shoulder blade to "wing out." A woman may notice that her arm feels weak when her hand is elevated to eye level, and that her shoulder blade feels as though it is sometimes out of place. This problem is almost always resolved by time alone, as the nerve wakes up and returns to normal function levels within a few weeks.

Rarely, a second motor nerve that connects the *latissimus dorsi* muscle with the brain can be damaged. This muscle lies on the back, below the shoulder blade, and helps to pull the arm backward. Loss of function of this muscle can contribute to weakness in certain arm functions. (See Chapter 6 on reconstruction for more on this).

Surgical Drains

At the end of all of these surgical procedures, the surgeon may place one or more porous drain tubes under the skin to allow fluid to drain off. Fluid continues to accumulate in the tissue for a few days because of the trauma caused by the surgery. The drain tubes are attached to a vacuum suction bulb that collects the fluid. While the woman is still in the hospital, the nurses teach her how to empty the suction bulb every few hours. Once she is proficient at emptying the bulb and can control her surgical pain with oral medication, she is ready to go home.

• • • Radiation

Radiation therapy is routinely prescribed for women who undergo a lumpectomy for a malignant tumor. This is necessary because lumpectomy alone does not guarantee that all cancer cells have been removed. Breast cancer cells can grow simultaneously in more than one location in the breast. Lumpectomy removes the primary organized tumor. Any additional colonies of cancer cells must be destroyed by radiation in order to remove the disease. This is why the two choices of surgical treatment offered to a woman to treat her disease are mastectomy or lumpectomy *with* radiation. Radiation may also be prescribed when a mastectomy is performed if the tumor is very large or if the tumor has invaded the chest muscle or armpit tissue.

• • • Out of the Hospital and Back Home

Once the drain tubes have been removed, a woman should begin to restore her shoulder motion so that she will be able to use her arm normally again. Following the lymph-node dissection, the patient is encouraged to use her arm by her doctors and nurses. She will need direction and guidance about how far to reach up, how long to hold the effort, and how much discomfort to expect. Physical therapists are the health professionals trained to provide this direction and guidance. They are available in hospitals, clinics, and private practices. If a patient's surgeon does not automatically refer her to a physical therapist at this point, she should request it.

Some women are able to reach straight up, behind their heads, and to the side without difficulty as soon as the drains are removed and their surgeon urges them to move normally. These women are able to return to their usual daily routine in two to three weeks. The majority of women, however, are not so fortunate. The first complication often begins to occur about a week after surgery. Sensations of burning, soreness, and tingling develop along the upper inner arm and on the outside of the chest wall. Rubbing the surface of the inner arm against the side of the chest adds to the discomfort. These hypersensitive sensations are similar to those you experience in your lips and cheek after receiving novocaine at the dentist's office. These surfaces are numb because nerves in the skin that supply sensation were cut during the operation. They revive and come alive during the second or third week following surgery. Women describe a variety of sensations:

"The inside of my arm feels sunburned."
"Someone took sandpaper to my skin."
"I have a baseball in my armpit."
"It feels like a vise around my chest."

These sensations of irritation and pressure are normal and to be expected. They intensify, peak, and then subside in the pattern of a bell-shaped curve. This whole process usually lasts two to six weeks, and averages three to four weeks. The active period of hypersensitivity, pain, and irritation fortunately runs its course and resolves with time. Many women, however, have patches of skin on the arm that remain permanently numb.

Even though the hypersensitive period is temporary, it does contribute to the loss of shoulder motion. Because the natural inclination is not to move your arm when it feels this way, you may find yourself walking around looking like Napoleon, holding your arm away from your side with your hand across your stomach. Too much of this habit encourages the surgical scar tissue to tighten and the tense muscles to shorten. This is particularly true if the surgery was performed on the left side and you are right-handed, or on the right side and you are left-handed. People naturally use their dominant arm spontaneously to reach for objects, open doors, feed themselves, or brush their hair. It becomes too easy not to move the arm that has been operated on if it is not the dominant arm. If you don't have to reach up or out with that arm, you won't.

Simultaneous to the hypersensitivity phase, a second sequence of events is going on. Since the lymphatic tubes or vessels that drain lymph out of the arm along its inner surface run directly through the armpit, many of these vessels were cut during surgery. They are too small to repair, and so the body is forced to compensate for their loss. After the axillary lymph-node dissection, there is often a residual fold in the skin that runs through the armpit and down the inner surface of the arm. In this skin fold are the superficial lymphatic vessels that have been damaged and can no longer carry fluid. As they dry up, these tubes shrink, which causes them to stand out like tight strings in the skin, and they often become sore and irritated. The sensation of them drawing tight may be felt clear down into the wrist. Some women discover that it is painful and very difficult to completely straighten their elbow.

A third possible complication is the tendency for the large chest muscle, the pectoralis major, to cramp and spasm. This can cause sharp, intermittent pain across the front of the shoulder and chest wall. However, this pain can often be avoided. The muscle cramps because of the build-up of tension from holding your arm too still and not moving it normally. The sooner you stretch out your arm and reach for objects in the usual way, the less chance you will have of experiencing this type of pain.

The message here that bears repeating is that movement resolves most of these problems. The exercises outlined in the following chapters will tell you how and when to move your arm to get it back to normal.

Once in a while, shoulder pain and stiffness can progress into inflammation and scar formation in the tissue around the shoulder joint, causing *adhesive capsulitis,* or "frozen shoulder." This means the shoulder tightens up so much that a woman cannot raise her arm above her head because the joint membrane or capsule has become scarred. The inflammation usually starts in the shoulder tendons of the rotator cuff and spreads to the tissue below. There is a great deal of aching in the shoulder and upper arm in the early stages of frozen shoulder. It takes several weeks or months to resolve this problem and it usually requires intensive physical therapy.

••• Lymphedema

Every woman who has had breast cancer surgery that includes an axillary lymph-node dissection must also know about the possibility of swelling in the arm, called *lymphedema*. Ask your surgeon to explain lymphedema to you and to tell you how to help prevent it. It is important to understand the relationship between infection and swelling, which is described in detail in Chapter 7. Soon after having a lymph-node dissection, your surgeon, a nurse, or physical therapist should give you a list of skin-care precautions designed to prevent infection. These precautions are important for preventing breaks in the skin on the hand or arm on the side of your surgery, which might invite infection. You should also learn how to recognize and seek treatment for infection in the arm, a condition called *cellulitis*. Once you are familiar with this vital preventive information, you are much less likely to develop lymphedema.

• • • Reconstruction

Women who have reconstructive surgery at the time of their mastectomy may have additional problems. Whether they choose to have breast implants or tissue transplants, a delay in the surgical-wound healing sometimes occurs. If the reconstruction is done with transplanted tissue from another part of the body, the circulation in that tissue is temporarily fragile. Tiny blood vessels that were moved or disturbed take some time to reestablish themselves, which can prolong the closing of the incision. These women will also have another incision, on their back, abdomen or buttocks, that needs to heal.

Women who choose an internal implant for their reconstruction have a temporary expander (a balloon-like sack) placed under the chest muscle to stretch the tissue to form a breast mound and create a pocket for the permanent implant. Sometimes the expander is itself the permanent implant. When the expander is injected with fluid (usually sterile saltwater), the chest muscle may react by tightening and becoming very painful, limiting the ability to move the arm. Any women who has had reconstruction and who experiences difficulty in moving her arm needs to be doing a shoulder-exercise program as soon as her surgeon says the skin is ready for stretching.

• • •

There is good news: each of the conditions described here can be resolved. The following chapters describe the pattern, treatment, and resolution of each potential complication. Becoming familiar with these potential aftereffects *before* they occur can help prevent them from prolonging your recovery. At the very least, knowing what to expect will reduce your anxiety, prepare you to get the appropriate information, and help you to know when professional help is needed.

Getting Started with Basic Stretches

Vivian came in for physical therapy two and a half weeks after having a modified radical mastectomy. Vivian was a short, slender woman with delicate features and a shy smile. She looked younger than her age of 63. She was right-handed and the surgery had been performed on her left side. Her discomfort was immediately obvious because she held her left arm across her abdomen in the familiar Napoleonic posture. Since this was her nondominant arm, I knew we would have to work a little harder.

Vivian's hospital stay had been typical for her type of surgery. With modified radical mastectomy, a woman can usually expect to be home from the hospital in one to three days. If she has tolerated the general anesthesia well, is able to control the surgical pain with oral medication, and knows how to manage the drain equipment, she is ready to continue her recovery at home. She may still have a bandage over the healing wound, which is a linear incision about eight to ten inches long; the incision is usually horizontal across the chest but may be diagonal, angling downward from the armpit. She will also have one or more suction drain bulbs or vacuum containers attached to drain tubes that were placed under the skin at the time of surgery. She is taught how to empty the drain bulbs by the nurses at the hospital. The drain tube is usually removed by the surgeon during the first office visit a woman makes after her surgery, or whenever the fluid has stopped draining. Once back in her own familiar environment, she can gradually begin to restore her ability to reach for things and use her arm normally.

For many women, one of the more puzzling and unexpected complications of regaining full use of their arm is the restriction of the skin under the arm. An axillary lymph-node dissection diminishes the elasticity of the skin under the arm. Because an oval-shaped section of skin on the breast containing the nipple was removed (the nipple cannot be saved because it could easily contain cancer cells), there is less skin to pull together to close the incision. It is as though a tuck in the skin on the chest was taken when the incision was closed. Also, lymph vessels that lie close to the skin on the undersurface of the arm had to be cut so that lymph nodes could be removed. After surgery, they shrink and become taut, and are often very sore. These vessels, which now act like thin bands of scar tissue, resist being stretched to their full length. The combination of less skin on the chest and tightness under the arm makes the simple act of raising the arm painful and difficult.

Vivian and I began the task of restoring her physical mobility. I had her lie down on her back on the treatment table. We spent the next several minutes practicing a simple breathing technique, borrowed from natural-childbirth training, which teaches a woman to breathe deeply and to blow out slowly through pursed lips. Learning to master long, slow, expirations and deep inspirations helped Vivian to relax and focus on the task. The breathing distracted her from the pain, and established a natural rhythm for the movement of the exercise. "Deep Breathing" is the first and perhaps most important exercise to master in this book.

"I want you to be able to blow out steadily for five seconds, then close your lips and breathe in through your nose naturally," I told her. "It should take you twice as long to blow out as it will take to breathe in again. When this rhythm feels natural, repeat the cycle three times in succession."

At first, Vivian could not get the air out very well. When a person is in pain or is anticipating pain, she naturally tends to hold her breath or take very shallow breaths. But this intensifies both the discomfort and the anxiety.

I coached Vivian to use her imagination and powers of concentration. "Visualize a candle two feet above your face. Now blow it out slowly. Push the air out using your diaphragm. Purse your lips to force the air out of your cheeks.

"Using this breathing technique will help you feel in control when you do add the stretches. Each time you blow out, you will stretch your arm a little further. Each stretch will last as long as it takes you to breathe in and out three times."

When she mastered the breathing, we added shoulder motions. Overhead elevation is the key motion to restore first, because other shoulder motions come back more easily once the ability to reach up has been recovered. I handed Vivian a wooden dowel rod about 24 inches long and 1 ½ inches in diameter, and taught her how to do the "Overhead Reach" stretch.

"Hold onto this rod with both hands. Bring your knees up so your feet are flat on the table and your back has good support. Start with the rod right up over your face, and keep your elbows straight. Now as you blow out, slowly pull the rod back overhead. Relax your left [the operated-on] arm. Let your right arm and gravity do the work. When you do this stretch at home, you can use one of the extension tubes from your vacuum cleaner for the rod. It's lightweight and just the right size."

Vivian repeated this exercise three or four times. Each time she was able to go back overhead a little further. In less than 15 minutes, she had increased her ability to reach back overhead by 50 percent. I could see the tension drain out of her face. She looked at me and said: "This is the first time in two weeks that I don't feel helpless anymore."

Next, Vivian was to learn the "Butterfly Stretch"—how to bring her hands up behind her head, clasp her fingers together, and push her elbows down to the table. Restoring this motion allows Vivian to get her hand up to her head, necessary for styling her hair and for dressing. This motion is particularly difficult because the pectoralis major muscle is often tight and in a state of spasm. It is also the position where the skin under the arm containing the taut lymphatic vessels is in the tightest position. Because of its difficulty, the "Butterfly Stretch" requires patience, discipline, and good breathing technique. After a few minutes of concentrated effort, Vivian was able to bring her hands up and down from behind her head, which had been impossible for her a half hour ago.

For the next exercise, Vivian sat in a chair to learn how to do the "Side-Arm Stretch." I positioned her in front of a mirror so she could watch herself and not "cheat." For this stretch, she grasped the hand of her operated arm with her other hand and placed both hands on top of her head. She then pulled the hand of her operated arm up over the top of her head, bringing her upper arm close to her ear. She laughed at herself as she saw that she was moving her head toward her arm instead of her arm toward her head.

"That happens a lot," I laughed with her. "Our bodies are famous for finding the easiest way."

Vivian rested and lowered her arms between efforts. Each repetition was a little easier to do; by the fifth time, she was able to bring the upper part of her arm to within two inches of the side of her head.

"Be sure to relax your left arm," I reminded her. "It's just going along for the ride. The right arm should be doing all the work."

The last exercise for Vivian was to stand up and "climb the wall." Facing the wall and using her new breathing technique, Vivian was able to reach well up over her head. Each time she blew air out, she stretched up higher. When I told her to look up and compare her two hands, she was surprised to see how far up the left one was able to reach.

We stopped at this point because I knew that these four stretches would be enough for Vivian to work with for the next few days. It is important not to start out with too many exercises; it is much better to be successful with a small program than to be overwhelmed by a lengthy one.

As I gave Vivian an illustrated page of instructions for these exercises, I told her she should repeat each exercise five times and hold each individual effort as long as it took her to complete three breathing cycles. If she was unable to get through five repetitions, she could start with three and then add one more each day until she was up to five. She was to do all four stretches twice a day, which would take her only 10 to 15 minutes to complete the program each time. A good routine to establish is to do the exercises after breakfast and after lunch. Bedtime is not a good time, since the body is tired, and the exercises are harder to do then. Vivian, like most women, could expect shoulder mobility to return in two to three weeks.

On her first visit, I noticed that the skin on Vivian's chest above and below her mastectomy scar was tight. I addressed this problem during her next treatment session, three days later. After reviewing the four stretches Vivian had been doing faithfully at home, I sat her in front of the mirror to teach a technique called *skin mobilization,* which helps to soften and loosen the skin on the chest wall. Vivian learned how to place the flat surface of the first three fingers of her opposite hand on her chest, just above the incision. She made slow circular motions, pressing in and stretching the skin with a gentle, gliding force. She worked her way across the top, then back along the underside of the incision. She performed the slow, circular motion five times clockwise, then five times counterclockwise, each time placing her fingers at a new location. She was to perform this technique once a day at home, usually just after taking a warm shower. The moist heat would help to soften the skin and make it easier to move around.

Free movement of skin on the front of the chest is necessary for normal shoulder motion. After a mastectomy, the chest skin is more taut because a tuck has been taken. Skin tightness of this type is unique to a mastectomy. Unlike abdominal surgery, where the surgeon opens the skin and enters a cavity, the breast surgeon works in a horizontal plane between the skin and the ribs. After the incision is made, the breast tissue is removed from the underside of the skin by a scalpel or by electrocautery. Electrocautery is the use of an electrical current from a needle-shaped instrument that dissects the tissue away from the skin. When this technique is used, very little blood is lost; small blood vessels are sealed off by the electrical current as quickly as they are cut through. The surgeon removes a section of skin that is elliptical in shape and contains the nipple. After the breast tissue is removed and the lymph nodes and surrounding tissue are taken out of the armpit, the surgeon closes the horizontal or diagonal incision with sutures. The result is that the chest skin is stretched and sewn together over the flat, unyielding surface of the rib cage.

Fat serves as the body's lubricant. Everywhere in our body, layers of fatty tissue just under the skin help the skin to slide smoothly over muscles and joints whenever we move. When the fat is stripped away, as happens in a mastectomy, the skin heals by sticking down to the next layer of tissue, the *fascia,* or filmy tissue covering the chest muscle. Skin naturally slides horizontally, but scar tissue forms perpendicular to the tissue layers, causing the skin and underlying tissue to stick together. Some adherence is necessary for healing, especially during the first two weeks after the operation. If the skin adheres to the underlying tissue too long, however, it will not be able to slide and will begin to restrict arm motion. Skin on the chest must slide a considerable distance to allow full elevation of the arm. Doing the skin-stretch technique once a day helps restore elasticity to the area and makes mobility of the arm easier.

Vivian studied herself intently in the mirror as she proceeded with the exercise. As she practiced this technique, I could see she was becoming more comfortable looking at and touching herself. Many women find it difficult to accept the appearance of their surgical area. They are acutely aware that a valued part of their body has been permanently removed, and they may think of themselves as "disfigured." One of the best ways to resolve this feeling is to first take a good long look at it, and then to touch it. Touch is the language of acceptance. Accepting yourself as you are is an integral part of the healing process.

The last part of Vivian's treatment session was devoted to teaching her the skin-care precautions for preventing infection and swelling in the arm on the side of the surgery. I gave her a list and explanation of these precautions to read and memorize at her own pace (see pages 80–81). It should be *routine* for all breast-surgery patients who have had an axillary lymph-node dissection to be taught this vital, preventive information.

Vivian was very motivated to restore her normal movement and function. She understood the importance of doing her exercises regularly twice a day, and not overdoing them. She remained faithful to the program we had outlined together, and when I saw her again ten days from her first physical therapy appointment, she had regained 90 percent of her full shoulder motion. She reported that most of her pain was gone. She still noticed some leftover hypersensitivity in the skin on the underside of her upper arm, which she told me was improving each day.

I encouraged her to start shopping for a breast prosthesis. Vivian had just received a visit from an American Cancer Society Reach to Recovery volunteer, who was herself a recovered breast-cancer patient. From her own experience, the volunteer helped Vivian with many of her emotional concerns, and told her about the free services the American Cancer Society offers to breast-cancer patients, including a prosthesis display. I suggested Vivian schedule a trip to the local chapter office to see the display. This way, she could look at several different products without any sales pressure. I assured Vivian that she could begin wearing a prosthesis as soon as it felt comfortable to do so.

Vivian's recovery is typical of someone who gets the appropriate information about how to help yourself. She told me later that she had visited her surgeon and told him how helpful physical therapy had been, especially because it gave her the structure and guidance she needed for a successful recovery. She strongly expressed her hope that other women recovering from breast surgery would have the same opportunity.

••• How To Move Your Arm Again: Exercises and Illustrations

When you do the following exercises at home, find a quiet place where you won't be distracted. Wear comfortable clothing, such as a loose-fitting cotton shirt and sweat pants, shorts, or a full skirt. Try to avoid tight outfits that will bind you in the middle.

Carpeting or a padded rug are best for the lying-down exercises. If it is not easy to get down on the floor, choose the bed with the firmest mattress and place your head at the foot of the bed, away from any walls.

Do not bounce or jerk your arms when doing any of the stretches. The movements should be slow and smooth, as though you are performing a slow-motion ballet.

Most people do these stretches twice a day, before or after breakfast and lunch. Don't wait until the end of the day when you will be too tired to do a good job. Do the exercises in the following order; they are given names and numbers to help you keep track of them.

Exercise 1: Deep Breathing

Lie flat on your back with your knees bent, feet flat on the floor, and arms at your sides.

Breathe in slowly and deeply through your nose, with lips closed. Blow out slowly through pursed lips. Visualize a candle two feet above your face and blow the flame out slowly.

Repeat the breathing cycle three times in succession. Then breathe normally for a few seconds. Practice the deep-breathing pattern a few times until you feel that you have a smooth rhythm. Then begin the stretches. You will use the deep-breathing technique during each stretch.

When using deep breathing while performing a stretch exercise, do the actual stretch (move your arms) during the expiration, or blowing-out phase. Hold your progress (don't move your arms) while you inhale again through your nose.

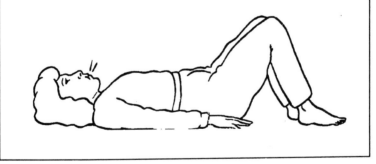

Exercise 2: Overhead Reach

Lie on your back with knees bent and feet flat on the floor. Hold onto a rod (such as a dowel, tube, or cane) with both hands. Have your hands as far apart as your shoulders (18 to 20 inches).

Raise the rod up over your face with your elbows straight. Slowly bring the rod back overhead, while blowing out through pursed lips. Have the unoperated arm do the pulling; the other arm should be completely relaxed. Move just a few inches, then hold your progress (don't move any further) while you breathe in through your nose. Blow out slowly while you advance the rod further back.

Each time you blow out and stretch further back should last about five seconds. If it is easier, you can count out loud to five by thousands ("a thousand and one, a thousand and two," etc.).

Repeat the breathing cycle three times, advancing the rod backward each time you blow out; then return the rod to the perpendicular position. To end the stretch, lower the rod all the way down by bending your elbows, and rest the rod on your abdomen.

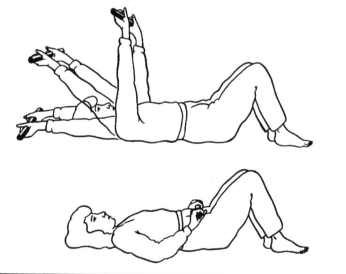

Rest briefly; then repeat the entire sequence three to five times.

Whenever it is easier or more comfortable, you can do the Overhead Reach stretch *without* the rod by just holding onto your wrist. The hand on the unoperated side holds the wrist on the operated side. Everything else about the stretch technique is the same.

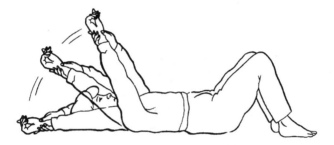

As you get stronger you may need more of a challenge. You can substitute a small, 1-2 pound weight for the rod and hold your wrist with the other hand. Be careful to keep your wrist straight and not overextend it backwards.

If you don't have a small weight, a household hammer is about the right weight and works well.

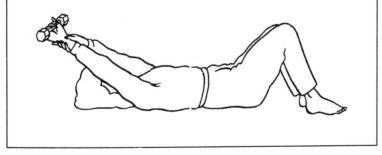

Exercise 3: Butterfly Stretch

Lie on your back with knees bent and feet flat on the
floor. Clasp your hands together loosely and place them
behind your head; keep both elbows close to your face.

Slowly lower your elbows down toward the floor as
you blow out through pursed lips (visualize blowing out
a candle).

Repeat the breathing cycle three times, pushing your
elbows lower each time you blow out. You will feel
tightness and pulling in the armpit and on your chest on
the operated side. Be sure to lower the elbow of the
other arm all the way to the floor.

To release the stretch, lift both of your elbows back
up to your face, unclasp the fingers and lower your
arms to your sides. Rest, and repeat the entire sequence
three to five times.

There are certain circumstances for which the "Butterfly Stretch" is not appropriate. If you have a history
of tendinitis or bursitis in either shoulder, this stretch

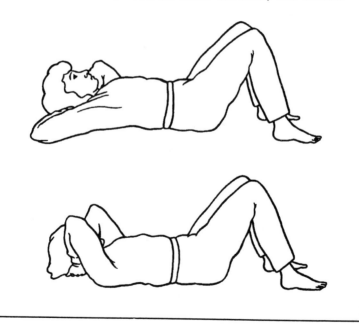

position may aggravate the condition. Tendinitis pain is commonly felt on the point of the shoulder and down along the *outside* of the upper arm, particularly when the arm is raised out to the side, or rotated outward. If the Butterfly Stretch position sets off this type of shoulder and arm pain, omit this exercise.

Exercise 4: Side-Arm Stretch

Do this exercise in front of a mirror, if possible.

Sit in a straight chair. Hold onto the wrist on the operated-on side with your opposite hand. Rest both hands on top of your head with your elbows pointed out to the sides. Keep your head up straight.

Slowly pull the arm on the operated side *toward* your head, as you blow out slowly three times. Try to get the upper part of your arm to touch your ear. Be sure you are not moving your head toward your arm.

Lower both arms; rest briefly, then repeat the entire sequence three to five times.

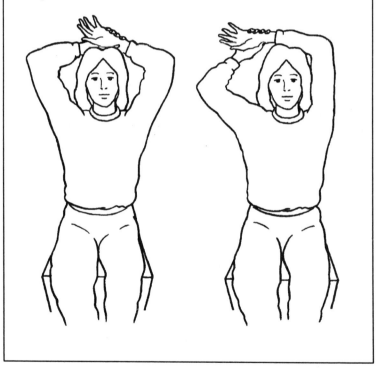

When you are able to do this stretch easily, increase the challenge by bending your torso to the side opposite the operation. Be sure not to lift your hip off the chair.

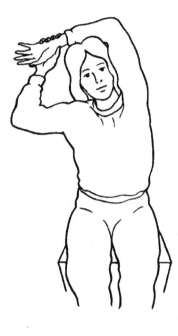

Exercise 5: Wall Climb

Stand facing the wall. Place your feet six inches back from the wall and rest your forehead on the wall for balance. Place your palms on the wall just above your head.

Begin to "walk" your fingers straight up the wall, advancing both hands up overhead each time you blow out. Walk the unoperated arm up until it is completely straight at the elbow. Then coax the arm on the operated side to go straight up as far as you can make it go.

Step backwards to lower both arms and rest. Repeat the entire sequence three to five times.

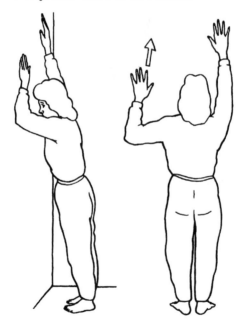

These are not the only exercises appropriate for restoring arm use after surgery for a mastectomy. Others described in the following chapters are also effective, depending on which motion or function you need to emphasize. For example, the "Buddha Stretch" in Chapter 4 is a favorite of many women.

Exercise 6: Skin Stretch

Sit facing a mirror. Place the hand on the operated side on top of your head. Place the flat surface of three fingers of the other hand on your chest just above the mastectomy scar line.

Press the skin against the ribs and move the skin in *slow* circular motions, five times clockwise, and five times counterclockwise. This is the same motion you use when doing breast self-examination, except that here you are pressing harder and making bigger circles.

Next, move your fingers along the scar one to two inches and repeat the entire sequence. Repeat the circular skin stretches across the top of the scar, and then back across the chest just below the scar.

Do this exercise once a day, preferably just after a warm shower.

Do not use skin lotion before doing this exercise because it will cause your fingers to slide around. Apply lotion to the chest area *after* doing the exercise if you want to keep the skin soft. Be sure the lotion does not get onto the incision itself if there are any open draining areas.

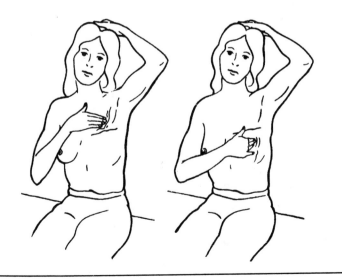

Preparing for Radiation

Terry began her physical therapy two weeks after having a lumpectomy and axillary lymph-node dissection. Terry was a tall woman in her late thirties, a loan officer at a local bank. She was scheduled to begin radiation treatments within the next few days, but it was a deadline both of us were concerned we were not going to meet.

Radiation therapy is necessary after a lumpectomy, even though the tumor has been removed, because there could be isolated groups of cancer cells elsewhere in the breast. The first part of the radiation-therapy process is the simulation, which is a scheduled outpatient appointment for planning the radiation treatments. During the simulation, precise measurements of the breast area are taken, and markings or small tattoos are placed on the skin by the radiation oncology team. The patient must lie very still, for up to an hour, on her back with her arm positioned out to the side and rotated up over her head. When I first saw Terry, she was barely able to hold this position for even a minute.

Terry had two problems. First, she was experiencing the most intense period of the skin hypersensitivity phase, which I call the "novocaine effect." During the first week after surgery, the skin of her upper inner arm was numb. Then, as feeling returned, she had predictable sensations of irritation and hypersensitivity. Now her arm felt sunburned and raw. The second problem was that she also had shortened, sore lymphatic vessels that caused a tightness in her upper inner arm. The sensations Terry was feeling are very common, and they could have resulted whether she had undergone a modified radical mastectomy or a lumpectomy. In either case, she would probably have had a lymph-node dissection, the surgery that causes these problems.

Terry is left-handed and the surgery was performed on her left side. She had not used her arm very much because the shortened lymphatic vessels from the armpit incision were so uncomfortable. By the time she came in, she was not able to straighten her elbow completely.

"The first thing we have to do is postpone your simulation," I suggested. "There is no way you could tolerate lying still with your arm out to the side until this pain is under control."

I contacted her surgeon and explained the situation. The surgeon called the radiation oncologist, who suggested the simulation be delayed for one week. This gave us time to improve Terry's arm mobility and to reduce her pain.

Even when Terry was lying down with her arm supported on a pillow, she was uncomfortable. Starting right in with the basic stretching exercises described in Chapter 3 would have been too painful. We needed something to relieve the pain enough so that she would be able to do the stretches effectively. *Ultrasound,* a form of electronic deep heat commonly used by physical therapists, was the solution.

I made sure that Terry was comfortable on the treatment table. I positioned her arm on pillows so that it was comfortably extended, with her palm up, and explained what to expect: "You will feel the light pressure of the applicator on your skin, and possibly a mild soothing warmth. The treatment is painless. I will keep the applicator in motion the whole time. I'm going to work on your upper arm, and along the inside of your elbow, where you see those tight lymph vessels that look like strings standing out in the skin. This will only take six minutes. All you have to do is lie there and think beautiful thoughts!"

Immediately after her first treatment, Terry felt a noticeable improvement. The tight lymphatic vessels running along the inner surface of her arm felt softer and more elastic. Right away, she was able to reach overhead more easily and with less discomfort. After several repeated attempts, she was able to get her elbow straight.

... Ultrasound, the Gentle Rescuer

Ultrasound is a form of deep heat. The machine is an electronic generator that transforms electrical current into mechanical vibrations at very high frequencies. These waves of energy are much higher than the human ear can hear (1 million cycles per second), which is why it is called *ultra*sound. When used in a pulsed mode with low dosage, these sound waves create a microscopic vibration in the cells that stimulates increased blood flow and tissue repair. The vibration dilates blood vessels, which flushes the area being treated with fresh oxygen and nutrients from the blood stream. This action soothes irritated and inflamed tissue, softens thickened tissue, and speeds up natural healing. It is used primarily to relieve localized pain in soft tissue.

Therapeutic ultrasound is related to but different from *diagnostic ultrasound,* which is a test used to study unborn fetuses, internal organs, even breasts. (Diagnostic ultrasound uses sound waves to create a computerized visual image of the object being studied.) Therapeutic ultrasound is administered by a hand-held, tube-shaped applicator, using a smooth continuous motion over the affected area. A water-soluble gel, which functions both as a lubricant and as a medium to conduct the ultrasonic waves, is applied to the surface of the skin over the area to be treated. The treatment lasts only a few minutes, and is painless. It has been my experience that patients who respond well to ultrasound for tight lymphatic vessels experience 70 to 80 percent improvement in both the pain and tightness after three to six treatments.

The ultrasound machine is about the size of a large shoe box and can easily be moved around on a small table with wheels.

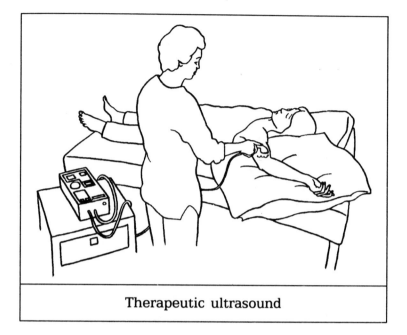

Therapeutic ultrasound

You should *not* have ultrasound treatments on an arm where you have had lymph-node dissection if you have any of these conditions: lymphedema, cellulitis (an active infection in the arm), or a history of or tendency to form blood clots in the arm. (See the section in Chapter 7 on lymphedema, page 76.) Ultrasound should not be performed over *any* area where there is a known tumor or suspected metastasis of tumor.

A scientific article published in January 1995 describes the effects of ultrasound on tumors in laboratory mice. The study concludes that ultrasound used in a *continuous* mode (which raises the temperature of the tissue) directly over the tumors, did cause the tumors to grow larger in treated mice than in untreated mice. No significant difference in metastases was noted in the two groups. The authors of the study suggest that the thermal effect of the ultrasound using the continuous mode heats the tumor and increases its blood supply, causing it to grow more rapidly.

Physical therapists and patients alike need to be aware of this new information, and to keep it in perspective. Ultra-

sound has been a valuable treatment used by physical therapists for the relief of pain for over 40 years. It is important that
the therapist uses ultrasound conservatively (for example, three
to six treatments, using pulsed mode and a low dosage). It is
also very important that the therapist knows the details of your
cancer diagnosis before using ultrasound. (See the Recommended Reading section at the end of the book for information on this study.)

Terry was a candidate for ultrasound on her arm. The pain
she was experiencing was preventing her from going on with
radiation therapy, which was a necessary part of her cancer
treatment.

After Terry's ultrasound treatment, she was ready to progress to the exercise program. Terry first learned the "Deep
Breathing" exercise (page 27). Then she tried the "Overhead
Reach" stretch (page 28). She was very apprehensive of the
pain, and was reluctant to apply enough pressure to get the
skin and lymphatic vessels to stretch. We needed to try other
methods. The most successful approach turned out to be the
"Buddha Stretch" (page 41). I had Terry get up on the table on
her hands and knees (all fours). From this position, I directed
her to slowly sit back on her heels, keeping her elbows
straight, and her hands flat on the table. She slowly lowered
her head between her arms as she lowered her body. This
position gives the appearance of "bowing to Buddha." Terry
felt the most in control when she was in this position. She was
successfully able to stretch both arms out straight in front of
her. She would release the stretch by returning to the all-fours
position. I had her repeat this motion slowly five times.

"There is something else I need to warn you about," I
added. "Sometimes one or more of these lymph vessels will
actually break while you are stretching your arm. No harm is
done. As a matter of fact, it is usually a relief. You will feel a
sudden 'ping' sensation in the arm, and then it will probably
feel looser. It's like breaking an adhesion (a band of scar tissue). Just go on with your exercises—they will probably be
easier to do."

Exercise 7: Buddha Stretch

Get down on the floor on your hands and knees (all-fours position). Spread your knees slightly for balance. Place your hands directly below your shoulders.

Slowly sit back on your heels and lower your head between your arms. Keep your elbows straight, and your hands flat on the floor. Hold this position as you blow out slowly three times.

Rest by returning to the all-fours position.

Repeat three to five times.

Move your hands forward two to three inches each time you repeat the stretch to increase the challenge.

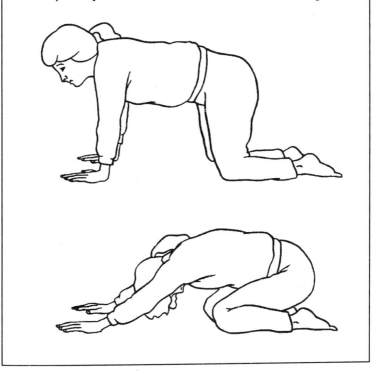

The "Buddha Stretch" gained enough flexibility for Terry immediately that, after several attempts, she was ready to lie on her back and do the "Overhead Reach." Next we worked on getting her hands up behind her head for the "Butterfly Stretch" (page 30). Once again it took several attempts with her concentrating on the breathing technique before she was able to comfortably get her hands behind her head with her elbows pushed back. After accomplishing this, she learned the "Side-Arm Stretch" (page 32). We decided to substitute the "Buddha Stretch" for the "Wall Climb" (page 34), because it worked much better for her.

By the end of the treatment session, Terry did each of these four stretches at least three times. She went home with written instructions, determined to make progress on her own before her next appointment two days later.

• • • Awakening Weakened Muscles

When she did return two days later, Terry was pleased with her progress but was also discouraged, because she thought it was taking longer than expected. She was anxious about delaying the radiation therapy. However, the radiation oncologist reassured her that one week was not a significant delay, and that her ability to maintain the position necessary for accurate measurements was very important. As the week progressed, Terry's mobility improved considerably, but some of her skin discomfort also increased. She was afraid that she was causing the problem, but I explained that this was not the case. The passage of time was causing her sensation to return, and she was entering the hypersensitive stage right on schedule. If anything, I told her, being able to concentrate on the exercises would probably help her tolerate this phase better.

Terry came in for treatment sessions every other day. By the third session, another problem needed addressing. Terry had a "winging" shoulder blade, which is caused by a temporary shutdown of the motoɪ nerve that controls the *serratus anterior* muscle, the muscle holding the shoulder blade close to the rib cage. (See Chapter 2, on axillary lymph-node dissection, page 12). This condition did not cause any pain; instead, it contributed to a feeling of weakness in Terry's arm whenever she tried to reach for an object in front of her, such as lifting a milk carton out of the refrigerator. This problem could just as easily have developed if Terry had undergone a mastectomy. We started working on two exercises to help this muscle regain its strength.

Exercises do not alter the pace at which nerves regenerate— the process by which they repair themselves with new nerve cells. Rather, time is their elixir. A muscle that is paralyzed by trauma to a motor nerve is not receiving messages from the brain through that nerve. But exercises help a paralyzed muscle "remember" how to work when the new nerve cells do reach it. The purpose of such exercises is to "talk to" the weakened muscle as it is returning to life. You communicate with a muscle by isolating and concentrating on the motion that is that muscle's particular job. For example, the biceps muscle bends the elbow and lifts your hand up. The serratus anterior muscle holds the shoulder blade next to the rib cage when your arm is elevated.

I had Terry lie down on her back on the treatment table with her knees bent. She raised her arm to the perpendicular position, so that her hand was directly over her face with her elbow straight. She then thrust her hand up toward the ceiling, pushing the arm upwards from the shoulder. The serratus anterior tries hard to work in this position if it can. She did not need to use the deep breathing technique this time, because this exercise is not a stretch and it is not painful. The "Shoulder Thrust" is an isometric exercise for muscle strengthening. (*Isometrics,* sometimes called contract-relax exercises, are static tension exercises in which you hold part of your body in a certain position or press against a resistance for a few seconds.) The muscle is working hard, even though there is no movement. When a muscle is challenged repeatedly, it gets stronger.

In the case of the "Shoulder Thrust," gravity is the resistance that creates the challenge.

Terry thrust her arm upwards and counted to five out loud by thousands ("a thousand and one, a thousand and two, etc."). By counting this way, she held the effort for five seconds, and kept breathing regularly. When she counted out loud, she had to breathe. She lowered her arm to rest, and repeated the exercise five times.

For the second strengthening exercise, Terry stood up, facing the wall. She placed her hands on the wall at shoulder height. She moved her feet back two feet and rested her forehead on the wall for balance. She then pushed herself away from the wall the same way someone does a push-up from the floor. The resistance was her body weight. Terry was soon able to do five "Wall Push-Offs" slowly and without difficulty. Later, we increased the challenge by having her do push-ups from her knees on the floor.

Terry liked doing the strengthening exercises. She said they gave her a new sense of power. She was asking her body to meet a challenge that required effort without pain. The "Wall Push-Off" exercise is a good one for anyone to do, whether or not you have had breast surgery, because it builds arm and upper-body strength without unnecessary strain.

• • • What to Expect from Radiation

Terry wanted to learn as much as she could about the radiation treatments. "What do your other patients experience when they have radiation?" she asked.

"The most common occurrence is skin irritation on the breast," I told her. "And that varies considerably. The skin gets red and may peel just like a sunburn. If it gets too bad, the technicians may stop the treatments for a few days and let the skin recover. After the treatments are finished, the redness and sensitivity usually disappear rapidly. There may be a change in pigmentation of the breast, usually darker, but this is often

Exercise 8: Shoulder Thrust

Lie flat on your back with knees bent and feet flat on the floor. Raise your arm to a perpendicular position, so it is straight up over your face.

Reach for the ceiling by thrusting the whole arm up from the shoulder. Keep your elbow straight. Hold the position while you count out loud to five by thousands. Lower the arm, and rest.

Repeat five to ten times.

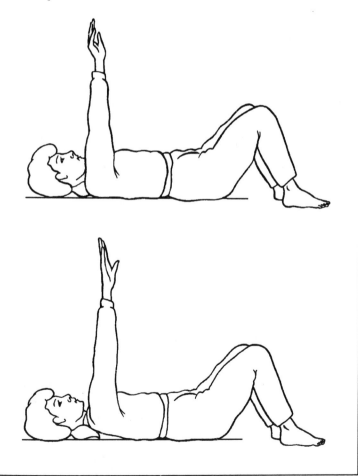

Exercise 9: Wall Push-Off

Stand facing the wall. Place your feet back about 24 inches and rest your forehead on the wall. Place both palms on the wall, level with your head.

Push yourself back away from the wall until your elbows are straight. Lower yourself slowly back to the wall.

Repeat this motion slowly five to ten times.

Be sure you are pushing from your arms, and not lifting yourself with your back. Your body weight is the resistance that makes your arms work hard. The further back your feet are, the harder your arms have to work.

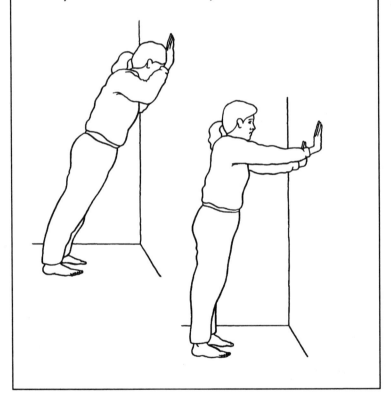

Exercise 10: Push-Ups from Your Knees

Get down on the floor on your hands and knees (all-fours position). Spread your knees for balance.

Lower your upper body and touch your nose to the floor. Then push yourself back up to the all-fours position with your arms. Be sure you are pushing your body weight up with your arms, and not lifting yourself with your back.

Repeat this motion slowly five to ten times.

This is a more challenging version of Exercise 9, the Wall Push-Off.

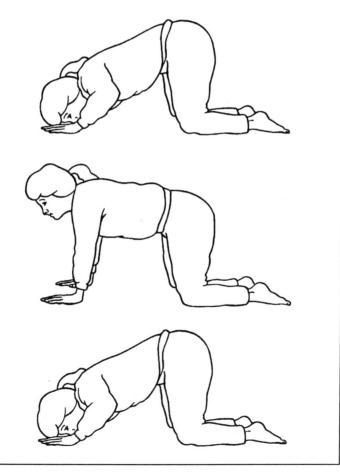

temporary. The breast will probably feel firmer for awhile, either because the skin is thicker or because the breast is swollen, or both. Much later, when all the reaction is over, the breast may be either larger or smaller than it was before treatment."

"Will the treatments make me sick?"

"No. That's because your digestive tract is not exposed. You may well notice some fatigue, especially during the last few weeks. Your body feels drained of energy because it is working hard to repair normal cells damaged by the radiation. It is also tiring just to get yourself into the hospital every day for the treatments. Just be sure you get enough rest and don't push yourself too hard.

"You will have to structure your day around the treatments. A schedule will be set up for you so that you can come in at the same time every day. You will probably get the weekends off, but your daily life will revolve around radiation therapy for the next several weeks.

"It is also important to keep up your shoulder stretches every day, even for a few weeks after the treatments have been completed, because radiation can cause the skin to tighten up and you could loose mobility. To kill the cancer cells, the radiation has to be strong enough, but it will also affect some of the normal cells in its path. Radiation can make the breast tissue harder and the skin less elastic because it causes an internal form of microscopic scarring called fibrosis."

Terry took all this in very pensively. I could see that she needed a plan of action to prepare for the simulation. We worked steadily on the exercises, and after four ultrasound treatments she felt she was ready. She did get through the procedure well and started her daily radiation treatments. I saw Terry once a week for the next three weeks to help keep the momentum of her shoulder exercises going. By the end of the fourth week of radiation, her motion and function level were back to normal, and she returned to work. Her supervisor was very supportive and allowed her to work a flexible schedule. By the time the radiation treatments were completed, she was able to handle a full day at work.

During her last visit, Terry told me how terrifying that early pain had been to her. She had felt so out of control and was afraid those feelings would never end. "I didn't know what was causing the pain, and I couldn't see an end to it. I grabbed onto those exercises like a drowning woman. They were something I could do for myself." If Terry had not responded so well to the ultrasound treatments, she might not have been able to start her radiation treatments for another two weeks or so. The time pressure probably turned out to be a blessing in disguise, because it spurred her to get the help she needed, and to find the determination to exercise diligently.

· · ·

Ultrasound, in addition to these exercises, is appropriate for a patient who is feeling pain and restricted arm motion during the first few weeks after axillary lymph-node dissection surgery, whether or not she is to have radiation therapy. Ultrasound is probably not necessary if eight to ten weeks have passed since the surgery, because the tight, painful lymphatic vessels will usually resolve themselves with time. Ultrasound speeds up the healing and reduces the pain, which is a large step in restoring arm function. (It is not, however, recommended for anyone who has lymphedema, cellulitis, a history of blood clot formation in the operated arm, or a known or suspected metastatic tumor.)

FIVE

What Can Happen
After an Implant

I was immediately impressed by Kendra's appearance. An attractive, well-dressed professional woman, she struck me as someone who is used to being in charge of any given situation. She was 47 years old, and had penetrating eyes and short hair. I recognized the familiar Napoleonic posture—she was holding her right arm across her abdomen—as a sign of her distress. I could see she was trying to conceal the pain she was feeling. I ushered her into the treatment room, told her how to get ready, and left the room. When I returned, Kendra was no longer trying to hide the pain. She sat hunched over in the chair, her arms folded across her chest. She opened the gown to reveal her reconstructed breast. Kendra had elected to have a simultaneous mastectomy and reconstruction with an implanted prosthesis. (Simultaneous mastectomy and reconstruction requires the teamwork of two surgeons: a breast surgeon first removes the breast, and a plastic surgeon then does the reconstruction. Both procedures are performed under one general anesthesia.)

At the time of Kendra's mastectomy three and a half weeks ago, the plastic surgeon had dissected the large chest muscle away from her chest wall and created a pocket for a temporary expander implant. He then placed the expander, a soft balloon-like sack with an outer silicone shell, in the pocket under the muscle on top of the ribs. During the few weeks following surgery, the expander would gradually be filled with saline (sterile saltwater). After Kendra's incision had healed, the surgeon began injecting saline directly into the expander to stretch the muscle and skin, creating a breast mound.

"I had my first expansion a week ago," Kendra said. "I guess I didn't know what I was getting myself into. I was doing really well up until then, and even started going back to my office. But after the expansion, the pain started. When my surgeon realized that it was getting steadily worse, he told me that I needed physical therapy."

In Kendra's case, the large chest muscle, the pectoralis major, was reacting strongly to the expansion. When the surgeon injected the implanted expander with saline, the muscle was passively stretched. The muscle was also still healing after having been separated from the ribs. The muscle reacted by going into an involuntary contraction or spasm, which was very painful and incapacitating.

Kendra's mastectomy incision was well healed and the skin above and below it was tight and shiny. I asked her to raise her arm up over her head. She made a valiant effort and got to just over shoulder height. It was the pain in the chest muscle that stopped her.

"I'm right-handed," she said, wincing and lowering her arm. "I can't go back to work like this!" There was a note of panic in her voice that surprised even her. "I've handled all of this pretty well until this pain. Now I feel as though it's all coming down on me at once." She couldn't hold back the tears any longer.

"That's good," I said softly, supplying a tissue. "You've probably been needing to do that for days."

"You're right," she answered with a weak smile.

In addition to the mastectomy and the implant expansions, Kendra was scheduled to begin chemotherapy the following week. Her apprehension was understandable; she was hardly ready to face another unknown treatment experience before she had her present situation under better control. I knew that Kendra needed some simple new techniques to teach her how to manage the pain. After an hour of work together, she would have those new tools.

As we talked, Kendra began to relax. I reassured her that what she was experiencing, both physically and emotionally, was not unusual under the circumstances.

I told her that one woman had described this pain as feeling as though she had a "bear trap clamped on her chest." Because Kendra didn't understand the pain in her chest, and didn't know what to do about it, her usual confidence was crumbling.

She climbed up onto the treatment table, lay down on her back, and began to learn the "Deep Breathing" exercise (page 27). I spent more time than usual making sure that Kendra really had the breathing technique mastered. She needed to learn to let her diaphragm do the work of breathing. This meant relaxing her chest muscles so that her chest would rise and fall in a natural rhythm.

Next, she started learning the first basic shoulder stretch, the "Overhead Reach" (page 28).

Kendra had a difficult time getting her arms back overhead. For Kendra to restore her ability to reach up with this arm, it would be important for her to first learn to move her painful arm passively, meaning she would learn to relax her right arm completely and have the left hand lift it back overhead (the left arm would be doing all the work).

Instead of having her hold onto a stick for the "Overhead Reach" stretch, I had her hold her right wrist with her left hand. She practiced holding both arms directly up over her face with the right arm *completely relaxed*. After she learned to raise and lower both arms this way (the left arm lifting and lowering the right one), she was able to begin slowly and gently stretching the right arm back overhead.

Because it is not easy to learn to relax a part of the body that is the source of pain, a person's natural instinct is to "protect the wounded wing" by tensing it. But this tension intensifies the involuntary spasm in the chest muscle. One more exercise would help relax Kendra's arm. I had her stand up and lean over, bracing herself on her left arm on the table. She dangled her right arm so that it hung down freely. She then learned to swing the arm slowly back and forth between her knees, in a loose, easy motion. This is "The Pendulum" (page 54). After a few minutes of practice, Kendra was able to swing her arm freely in four directions: back and forth, side to side, clockwise circles, and counterclockwise circles.

Kendra had accomplished the main goal of this first treatment session: learning tools she could use anytime to control the chest-muscle pain. Passive exercises like these gently move the muscle in spasm, which helps restore its circulation. Kendra also had to prevent her shoulder and elbow from becoming stiff, but she needed a few days just to concentrate on relaxing the tension and to master the passive movements. Letting some time pass would allow the pain to subside. We would go from there when she returned in a few days.

Kendra was visibly relieved when she returned later that week. She told me the pain was about 50 percent better. We reviewed her passive exercises, which she now did easily. The next step was to begin stretching the chest muscle and the shoulder itself. To stretch her *pectoralis major* chest muscle, Kendra would first have to learn how to alternately contract and then relax it. This technique would break the spasm and allow the muscle to return to normal. When the muscle became less irritable and did not spasm easily, Kendra would have an easier time with future expansions. She could use the following exercises to reduce the muscle tension after each expansion.

I had Kendra sit in a chair to learn some isometric exercises. She placed the heels of her palms together in front of her, just above her waistline, in a "praying hands" position. I then told her to press her hands together firmly, building up the pressure between her hands slowly, and count to five. At the end of the fifth count, she relaxed the pressure. She repeated the press and relax sequence five times. I call this exercise the "Chest Press" (page 55). Alternately contracting and relaxing the muscle in this manner helps to "flush" the muscle with a fresh blood supply and allow it to relax.

A muscle that is cramping continuously is literally not able to breathe. When it is contracting or knotting up, it squeezes

Exercise 11: The Pendulum

Stand next to the kitchen or dining room table (the kitchen counter is usually too high). Lean over at the waist and support yourself on your forearm (on the unoperated side) on the table. Bend over so that your back is parallel to the floor and your operated arm dangles perpendicular to your body. Spread your legs apart. Relax your arm so there is no tension in the arm or shoulder.

Swing the arm smoothly and freely back and forth between your legs ten times.

Now swing the arm from side to side in front of you (perpendicular to the first direction), another ten times.

Next, swing the arm in slow big circles, ten times clockwise and ten times counterclockwise. Stand up and walk around normally.

Repeat the sequence, ten times in each of the four directions, four to six times a day if you wish.

You can do the pendulum exercise frequently, any time your arm feels tense or you feel the need to move it. This exercise should not be painful. Expect to feel looser and more relaxed afterwards.

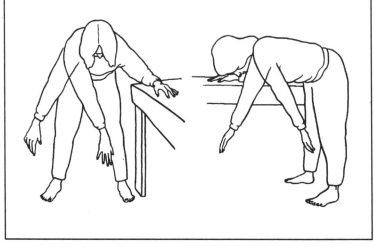

Exercise 12: Chest Press

Sit in a chair with good back support. Place the palms of your hands together directly in front of you, above your waistline. Your hands should be level with your elbows.

Press the heels of your palms together firmly as you count slowly to five, out loud. You will feel the effort in the muscles in the front of your chest. Then relax the pressure and lower your hands to your lap to rest.

Reposition your hands and repeat the press-relax sequence five times.

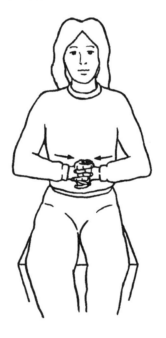

Exercise 13: Shrug-Relax

Sit in a chair with your arms straight down at your sides. Keep your back straight and your chin level.

Shrug your shoulders up toward your ears as you breathe in through your nose. Hold the shrug about three seconds. Then slowly lower your shoulders as you blow out through pursed lips.

Visualize blowing out a candle in front of you. Make the relaxation phase (blowing out) last twice as long as the shrugging up. A suggested rhythm is to breathe in and shrug up to three counts, hold three counts, blow out and lower shoulders to six counts.

Repeat the entire sequence three to five times.

You can do this easy tension-releasing exercise almost anywhere: sitting at a desk at work or even in the car waiting for the red light to change.

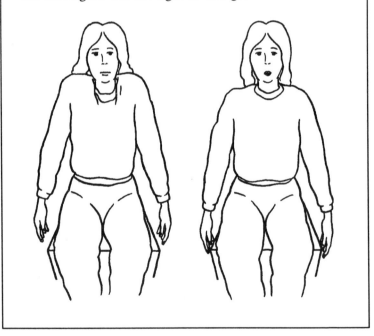

Exercise 14: Standing Chest Stretch

Stand facing a corner. Place one arm on each wall with your elbows level with your shoulders.

Slowly lean forward into the corner. Keep your knees straight and your feet flat on the floor. The closer you get to the corner, the more stretch you will feel in your chest.

Move forward and backward slowly at a pace that feels right to you. You can increase the challenge by moving your feet back.

Repeat the motion five times.

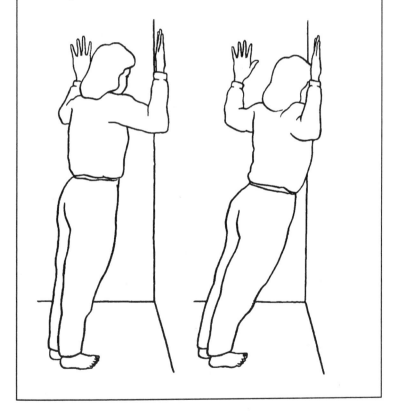

the tiny blood vessels (capillaries) that bring in fresh oxygen. Because the waste products of metabolism do not get flushed away, the muscle accumulates carbon dioxide and lactic acid, a by-product produced by burning glucose. Too much lactic acid causes muscles to become very sore and cramp even more easily.

I taught Kendra a second tension-relieving exercise called the "Shrug-Relax" (page 56). Still sitting in the chair, with her arms down at her sides, Kendra shrugged her shoulders up toward her ears. She held this position for a slow count of three, then slowly relaxed and lowered her shoulders. This exercise works well when using the deep-breathing technique. Kendra breathed in through her nose as she shrugged up and blew out slowly through pursed lips as she lowered and relaxed her shoulders.

I then added a third exercise, which was a gentle stretch called the "Standing Chest Stretch" (page 57). Kendra stood in the corner, facing inward, and placed one arm on each wall. With her elbows level with her shoulders, she slowly leaned forward lowering her chest toward the corner. In this position the pectoralis major muscle is stretched. This is a gentle stretch because it is easy to control the forward movement of the body with the legs. Kendra leaned forward and returned to her starting position slowly, five times.

As Kendra got ready to leave, she wanted to know how soon the pain in her chest and shoulder would be gone. I explained that women react very differently to breast implants and the expansion process. Some breeze through it with only fleeting discomfort. They may not need to do any exercises at all. Others are incapacitated for weeks and need physical therapy. In Kendra's case, she had accomplished so much in the first two treatment sessions that her prospects were very promising. I told her that having a second pair of hands to help her perform another exercise would be ideal. We decided to invite her husband, Gene, to her next session.

When they arrived two days later, Kendra introduced me to Gene. I could see he appeared somewhat uncomfortable being here, however, he obviously cared for Kendra and wanted to help if he could. I decided to put him to work right away; I asked him to slip off his jacket and roll up his sleeves. With Kendra on her back on the treatment table and Gene standing next to her, I demonstrated and coached them in a program of isometric exercises done with a partner (page 60).

Kendra began by pushing her arm against the resistance of Gene's open palm, which he placed at her elbow. It took several attempts for them to get the rhythm and pressure right. At first Gene tried to overpower Kendra. He had to learn to just meet her effort. I suggested that he set his body weight to be the resistance; he didn't have to push. She was in charge of how hard to push. Together they learned to time the efforts. She would breathe out slowly, he would count.

They alternated directions. First Kendra would press her arm up overhead, then down toward her feet. Each time, Gene applied resistance by switching his hand from one side of her arm to the opposite side, and held the effort for five seconds. Gene noticed that Kendra kept holding her breath.

"Kendra, why don't you do the counting. Count out loud to five by thousands, the way you did for your other exercises," I suggested. "If you count out loud, you have to breathe."

After completing this sequence five times each way, I demonstrated the same procedure, this time going across her body at a right angle to the original direction. Gene again applied the resistance at her elbow, alternating his resistance on each side of her arm.

"Think of your up and down presses as going north and south. The second series across your chest will be east and west. You will do these five times each way to wear the muscle out. When it is fatigued, the muscle will stop fighting, and you can stretch through the spasm."

They performed their isometrics against resistance in both directions, alternating pressure each way. As soon as they finished, I handed Kendra a two-pound hand weight. Still lying on her back, she held it in the hand on her operated side, and supported the wrist with her other hand (page 29). She slowly

Exercise 15: Partner Isometrics

Lie on your back on the bed or the floor, with your knees bent. Hold your arm straight up over your face (perpendicular to the floor), with your palm facing your knees.

Have your partner kneel next to you and place his or her open palm against your arm, just above the elbow.

Push against your partner's arm, toward your feet. Your partner should resist with equal pressure, so there is a strong effort but no movement.

As you push against the resistance of your partner's hand, count out loud slowly to five. Then relax the effort.

Next, have your partner switch his or her hand to the other side of your arm. Push up toward your head against the resistance. Count out loud to be sure you are breathing normally during the effort and to establish a rhythm for both of you.

Repeat these presses ten times, alternating directions five times each direction.

At the end of these isometrics, your shoulder muscles will be fatigued. This is a good time to stretch them, as they are less likely to resist. You can do this with the "Overhead Reach" (page 28), either with or without the rod, or by holding a small weight (one to two pounds) in your hand. A household hammer also works well.

After stretching, repeat the isometric presses with your partner, but this time at a 90-degree angle from the direction of the first set. Instead of pressing toward your head and knees, press to each side, alternating back and forth across your chest.

Have your partner place his or her hand on the inside and then the outside of your upper arm, close to your elbow.

Alternate directions, five times each way, for a total of ten times.

After completing ten resisted presses, do the "Butter-fly Stretch" (page 30).

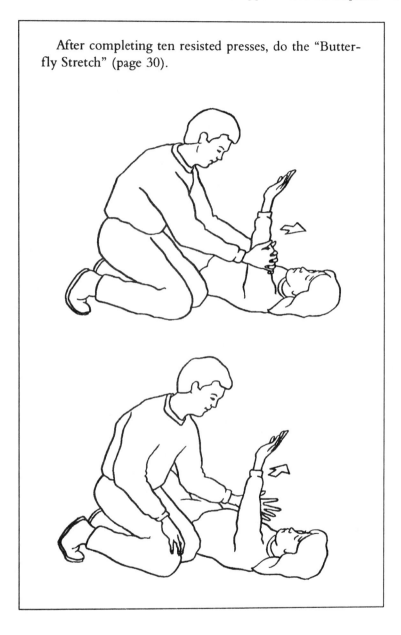

lowered the weight back overhead, stretching her reaching motion. This was the same stretch she had learned during her first visit, except that we now added the weight to increase the stretch. Then she did the "Butterfly Stretch" (page 30). Because the shoulder muscles were tired by the isometric efforts, there was much less resistance to the stretches.

When she finished, I saw the confidence in her eyes that I had glimpsed when we first met. She smiled and heaved a big sigh.

"I can do this," she said.

Gene was obviously more at ease also. After we talked for a few minutes, he said he had felt very helpless about Kendra's ordeal. He told me how frustrating it was to stand by and watch the person he loved suffer so much physically and emotionally, and not be able to stop it. Today's session had given him something *he* could do—now he felt as though he could be a part of Kendra's recovery.

Kendra went home with written instructions for her exercise program, a specific number of repetitions of each stretch to be done twice a day. She would also work with Gene on the isometrics at least once a day. The next time I saw her, three days later, she had achieved 75 percent of her normal shoulder mobility and the pain was 80 percent better.

"I wish I could tell you that this improvement level would last, but you must expect a little setback each time you receive an expansion," I told her. "The important thing is that you will know how to recover more quickly each time. Now that you know what to do and how to control the pain, you won't ever be in this much trouble again."

Kendra completed her expansions on schedule. She had four expansions, which is average; smaller-breasted women often need only one or two. Shortly after she finished her six months of chemotherapy, she was ready to undergo the final reconstructive surgery in which the plastic surgeon removed her expander and replaced it with a permanent prosthesis. This was done as an outpatient procedure under general anesthesia.

Kendra also decided to have nipple reconstruction, an optional procedure. Some women decide to go ahead with it when the expansions are completed; others are happy with the shape of their new breast and don't want to have any more surgery. For the nipple reconstruction, Kendra had to wait for the new incision from the placement of the permanent implant to heal (the surgeon had gone through the old mastectomy scar). There were several ways to create a new nipple from Kendra's own tissue. She chose to have some skin taken from her inner thigh. The surgeon grafted the section of skin to her breast and shaped it like a nipple. Later as an office procedure with local anesthetic, the surgeon tattooed on the areola (the pigmented area around the nipple).

Two weeks after her last operation, Kendra stopped in to see me and show off her finished reconstruction. She was celebrating the completion of her chemotherapy and the end of her surgeries. She had fully recovered her shoulder motion and the pain was gone.

"I have come through one of the worst times of my life," she told me. "I've had so many powerful and important feelings. I've learned more about how I can handle pain than I ever wanted to know. The day I took my last chemotherapy pill, I felt an incredible mixture of relief and power. I was also afraid, because you feel safe while you're on the treatments. I will never feel the same about what is really important again. My life looks very different to me now. I've learned that it's not as important to focus on whether the cancer comes back as how I live my days."

Partner isometrics can be performed in the same manner whether you have had a lumpectomy or mastectomy, with or without reconstruction. If you do not have chest muscle-spasm pain but want to strengthen your chest and shoulder muscles, this is an effective way to do it.

Any person can be a partner when you do these exercises at home. A partner can be your best friend, sister or brother, mother or daughter—not just a spouse. Many single women go through the recovery from breast surgery, but they are not alone; they have important people in their lives who are very concerned about their recovery. Choose as a partner someone who is interested in helping you, and who is easygoing and patient. You don't want someone who will overpower you or be too critical of your ability.

If you had a modified radical mastectomy months or even years ago and are now considering having an implant, you will probably not have as many problems as someone who has immediate reconstruction. This is because you have already recovered from your axillary lymph-node dissection. Remember, it is this surgery that causes so many of the problems that prolong recovery. As long as the original surgery left you enough skin to stretch over an implant, your recovery could be relatively uneventful by comparison. On the other hand, you may well have the same reaction in the chest muscle that Kendra experienced. If so, the exercises in this chapter are appropriate for you.

What Can Happen After a Tissue Transplant

Because of recent safety concerns about silicone gel-filled implants, breast reconstruction that uses transplanted tissue is being more frequently chosen by breast cancer patients. Such a transplant involves moving a woman's own tissue (muscle, fat, skin, and blood vessels) from some other part of her body to make a new breast after a mastectomy has been performed.

A few years ago the latissimus dorsi muscle flap procedure (called the *Latissimus flap*) was frequently performed. This wide, flat muscle lies on the back of the rib cage below the shoulder blade. It is transferred to the front of the chest, along with the blood vessels that nourish it, to create a breast mound. The muscle and blood vessels are rotated and tunneled under the skin on the side of the chest under the arm. Because there usually isn't enough tissue to create a breast mound equal in size to the remaining breast, the surgeon often needs to place an implant under the transplanted muscle. This procedure leaves a fairly long scar across a woman's upper back, with some residual weakness around her shoulder blade because the muscle was moved. This weakness is not usually noticeable unless she is an athlete and her dominant arm is affected. Performance in such sports as tennis or golf, for example, may be diminished. Fortunately, other shoulder blade muscles adjacent to the latissimus dorsi work in a similar way. Women who choose this procedure will also usually have an implant in their new breast (possibly preceded by an expander). The necessity of an implant and the surgical scar on the back have made the latissimus flap procedure less popular now than it was 10 to 15 years ago.

More recently, the *TRAM procedure* (which stands for transverse rectus abdominus myocutaneous flap), also referred to as the reconstruction with the "tummy tuck," has become the more popular choice. As with implant reconstruction, two surgeons work together if the transplant reconstruction is to be done simultaneously with the mastectomy. The breast is removed by the breast surgeon, then the plastic surgeon begins the reconstruction by making a horizontal incision across the lower abdomen, dissecting a layer of fat and skin and detaching part of the vertical abdominal muscle along with the blood vessels that feed this tissue. A portion of this tissue is transplanted to the mastectomy site and molded into a breast. The result is a soft mound with an oval-shaped scar across it, a horizontal abdominal scar from one hip to the other, and a flattened lower abdomen.

There are two types of TRAM flap procedures: free flap and pedicle flap. In the first, tissue is completely removed from the body before it is reattached. This is a more time-consuming procedure because the surgeon has to reattach several small blood vessels at their new location, which requires very intricate and delicate microsurgery, and may take as long as 8 to 12 hours. Fewer plastic surgeons have extensive experience with this procedure. In the pedicle-flap procedure, the blood vessels are not detached. Instead, the muscle, fat, and abdominal skin, along with their blood vessels, are rotated up through a tunnel created under the midriff area and are shaped and sewn in place as the new breast. This surgery is likely to take about four to six hours.

An alternate location for donor tissue is the buttocks area; this procedure is called a *Gluteus flap,* and is not common. This is also a free-flap procedure, where muscle, fat, and blood vessels are completely detached from the buttocks and reattached as the new breast. Just as with the free TrAM flap, this procedure requires microsurgery. The patient is left with a scar and possibly a flattened area on the buttocks. Latissimus flaps and Gluteus flaps may be chosen by women who cannot have either type of TRAM flap because of prior abdominal surgery and scar tissue, or because they are too thin.

Kate came to see me for physical therapy after reconstruction and had a complex combination of problems. She chose to have a modified radical mastectomy and a pedicle TRAM flap done simultaneously, all under one general anesthetic. Kate was 55 years old, medium height, and had a stocky, athletic figure. When she prepared for her surgery, she asked a lot of questions and looked at pictures supplied by the plastic surgeon. She knew the surgery would take many hours, but she made up her mind quickly and went ahead with the procedure.

When Kate came in for her first appointment after the surgery, she told me she wished she had taken more time to talk with other women who had undergone TRAM flap procedures. It is rigorous: this surgery can be compared to undergoing a hysterectomy, the removal of a gall bladder, and a mastectomy all at once. Two large incisions must heal, and part of a major muscle has been detached and moved. Occasionally, tissue-transplant patients have complications with wound healing. The skin may break down because it lacks adequate circulation. A woman may have to deal with a "weeping" wound and daily dressing changes for a few weeks after the surgery; other operations are sometimes needed to clean out or "debride" the healing area.

Kate was eager to get back to normal, and wanted to return to her position as an office administrator as soon as possible. But three weeks after her surgery, she still could not stand up straight. The only way she was able to sleep comfortably was in a recliner. She had had trouble with low back pain off and on before the surgery, but she did not think her back would act up after her surgery. But it did. Because of the abdominal incision, she was not able to stand up or walk straight, which aggravated her back. Her breast incision was open and draining because some of the skin had not healed, and she was changing her own dressings. When Kate realized that her pain and ability to move around were getting worse instead of better, she asked her surgeon to refer her to a physical therapist.

We had two problems to solve: restoring her shoulder function and resolving her back pain. The two incisions on her skin would heal at their own pace and would not interfere with our program. First, we went to work on the basic shoulder exercises. In the first treatment session, Kate learned the five basic exercises (in Chapter 3). She was right-handed and the surgery was on her left side. Fortunately, she had minimal movement restriction under the left arm from the axillary lymph-node dissection. Even though the breast incision was still open and draining, she needed to get going on her exercises before her shoulder started to stiffen. The open wound did not cause any additional pain; in fact, this area is usually numb. When some of the skin around the incision "dies" because the re-routed blood supply is still reestablishing itself, the wound then heals from the bottom up. New cells are formed until the opening fills in from below. For this reason, reaching motions and stretches do not interfere with the healing.

Kate, like everyone who has a lymph-node dissection, was experiencing the funny feelings along the upper inner side of her arm that I call the novocaine effect. Once she understood these uncomfortable sensations, she was able to focus her attention on the shoulder stretches. Learning the five basic exercises was enough for her to absorb in the first session. I anticipated that she would recover her shoulder mobility in the usual amount of time, about two to three weeks.

During Kate's second physical therapy session a few days later, we reviewed her shoulder exercises. She had already made excellent progress with improving her ability to reach up and overhead. Now we were ready to address the back pain. This meant designing a program of specific exercises to gently stretch out her abdomen, strengthen her back muscles, and restore her posture. Just being able to lie on her stomach over some pillows was difficult for her. After TRAM-flap surgery, some woman are not able to do this for several weeks. Because Kate now had sufficient upward-reach motion in her arm, she was ready to try to lie down on her stomach.

We overlapped two thick, soft pillows on the treatment table. Kate got onto the table on all fours and then slowly lowered herself down onto the pillows, which were positioned under her chest and abdomen. She rested her forehead on a rolled towel, so that her face was straight down and she could breathe easily. Her first back exercise, called the "Opposite Arm and Leg Lift" (page 70), was to learn to raise one arm and the opposite leg to build tone in the back muscles. She alternated the movements and held each one for five seconds in a pattern similar to swimming on dry land. Even though she was barely able to lift her left arm off the table, she could feel the effort in her back muscles where she needed it. She was able to lift each pair three times, quite an accomplishment for the first time she tried lying on her stomach.

For the second back exercise, Kate needed to get into a position that would stretch her abdomen and the lower part of her spine. With a little coaxing, she raised her chest up off the pillows and braced herself on her elbows, as though she were on the floor reading the newspaper. In this position, I had her breathe in slowly through her nose, and then blow out through pursed lips for five seconds. Each time she did the blowing-out part of the breathing cycle, I had her relax her back and let it sag like an old hammock.

This "Back Stretch from Elbows" exercise (page 71) is held in position for a few seconds; the position itself does the stretching. Kate could feel the stretch in her abdomen, especially around the incision, as well as in her lower back. Her abdominal incision was completely closed and well healed, and her belly skin was now ready to be stretched so that she could stand up straight.

Kate's third back exercise was "The Bridge" (page 72), performed lying on her back with her knees bent and her arms

Exercise 16: Opposite Arm and Leg Lift

Lie face down on the floor with pillows under your abdomen and chest. Rest your forehead on a rolled towel so that you can breathe easily through your nose. Extend your arms out overhead.

Lift one arm and the opposite leg and hold this position for five seconds. You do not need to lift them very high, just so they are up in the air. Count out loud so you do not hold your breath.

Rest; then repeat with the opposite pair.

Alternate the pairs five times each, counting to five out loud each time.

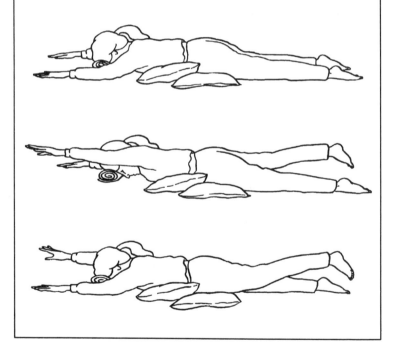

Exercise 17: Back Stretch from Elbows

Lie flat, face down, on the floor if possible, or on a firm mattress. If necessary, place pillows under your chest and abdomen. Prop yourself up on your elbows, as though you are going to read a newspaper spread out on the floor. Your upper body should be braced on your forearms. Be sure your elbows are directly below your shoulders.

Take a deep breath in through your nose. Slowly blow out through pursed lips and let your back sag. Be sure your trunk is completely relaxed. Repeat this breathing cycle three times, then lie flat again.

Repeat this entire sequence three to five times.

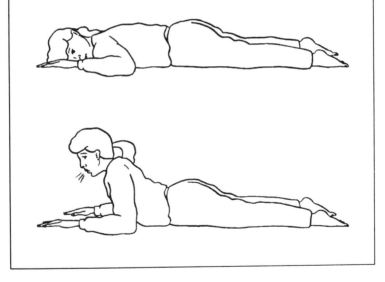

Exercise 18: The Bridge

Lie flat on your back, with knees bent, feet flat on the floor, and arms at your sides.

Raise your hips up in the air, so there is a straight line from your chin to your knee caps. Keep your head and shoulders flat on the floor. Hold this position and count out loud to five. Lower your hips to the floor and rest.

Repeat the lift five times.

You can do these exercises once or twice a day, as it feels best to you.

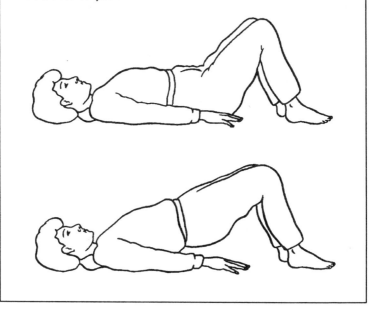

down at her sides. She pushed her hips up in the air until her body was in a straight line from her chin to her knee caps. Her head and shoulders remained flat on the table. Since this is a strengthening exercise, Kate felt effort but no pain. When she raised her hips all the way up, she counted out loud to five, by thousands, so that she held the effort five seconds and did not hold her breath.

Low back pain has multiple causes. In Kate's case, it was set off by the bent-forward posture—which was a direct result of the surgery. This posture, in turn, created muscle tension and stress. If she had had a spinal-disc injury or a condition called *spinal stenosis,* these exercises might not have been appropriate for her. If she were experiencing sciatic pain (nerve pain in the leg), the exercise program would have been different. Back pain that stays at the waist level or above is more often related to muscle strain. This kind of pain feels more like sore, cramping back muscles and is directly affected by changes in position: worse when standing or walking and better when sitting or lying down. It will often improve with the application of local heat, preferably moist heat, and nonprescription anti-inflammatory medication.

Even with her progress on the stretching exercises, Kate was distressed by the amount of time and energy she had to devote to her recovery. Her chest wound was slow to heal and required a daily changing of gauze bandages to absorb the wound drainage. She needed to work on her shoulder, abdominal, and back exercises twice a day. During her third treatment session, she realized how much time she might have wasted if she had not known what to do to help herself. But even so, she was frustrated that she ran out of energy so easily.

"Think of yourself as a fuel tank," I suggested. I drew a diagram of a tank with a faucet on each side to emphasize my point.

"Here is the faucet that dispenses your daily energy supply. The problem is that there is a second faucet dripping fuel continuously. This fuel is energy your body uses just to heal itself. When it is two o'clock in the afternoon, you think you have

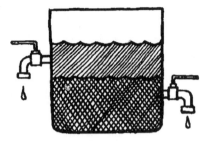

this much energy." I drew a line designating the tank's contents. "But actually, you only have this much." I drew a second line, lower than the first. "That's when you feel as though someone has pulled the plug on you. You suddenly feel very tired and probably not very tolerant of small irritations. Trust your body to tell you what it needs. When it says rest, go lie down. Your body will never lie to you; it will always tell you the truth. The challenge is learning how to interpret its messages. I believe this is one of the positive benefits of experiencing any illness or injury. You can learn so much by listening to your body."

Determination and perseverance paid off for Kate. Three weeks after beginning physical therapy, she was able to use her left arm for most of her daily activities.

After she was able to stand and walk straight, I taught her basic body mechanics to protect both her abdominal incision and her back. When she had to sit for long periods, she used a foam rubber roll or small pillow to support her lower back. She also discovered that she preferred a straight chair with arms rather than a soft, deep sofa. She learned the correct way to lift light objects from low surfaces by facing the object squarely, keeping her back straight, and bending from her knees. It was several months before she was allowed to lift anything heavier than a few pounds. Because she had some of her abdominal muscle removed, a sudden, forceful lifting effort could cause an abdominal hernia. Some women find it is very helpful to wear an elastic abdominal binder for a number of weeks after the surgery to give them support.

In addition to restoring her mobility and posture, Kate now knew that the back exercises and posture training would help to protect her from recurrent episodes of back pain. She also had a deeper appreciation and respect for her body. She understood how to handle pain more effectively. She had new information that would serve her for the rest of her life.

Kate thought hard about having nipple reconstruction. After the breast incision finally healed, she decided she had had enough of operations and healing wounds. She was very happy with the shape and feel of her new breast, and that was good enough for her.

When she stopped in for a brief visit a year later, Kate told me how she felt, looking back on the whole experience. She remembered at the time how she thought the pain and distress would never end. In hindsight, she said that even though she had not fully realized what she was getting herself into, the experience of being temporarily disabled and facing a life-threatening disease had taught her some valuable lessons.

"Now I know things about myself that I would never have learned any other way. I've learned to be a lot more tolerant of situations that used to frustrate and irritate me so easily. I think I'm more patient with life in general, because I know that everything can change so quickly without warning."

She was also very pleased with her reconstruction. "I can wear anything I want to," she smiled. "No one can tell which breast I lost. And best of all, there's nothing artificial. It's all me!"

Preventive Measures

One of the unexpected benefits of having to face a life-threatening disease is that it can teach you how to take better care of yourself. It is easy to take your health for granted when there is nothing wrong. The other extreme is to become obsessed with your body because of a health crisis. A happy balance is to be informed and vigilant. This chapter is designed to help you achieve this balance—to maintain your health and your peace of mind. The topics covered here are preventing infection and swelling in the operated arm, practicing breast self-examination, and knowing how to interpret new symptoms. Taking better care of yourself means practicing good health habits consistently, and directing your team of physicians to work on your behalf.

· · · Lymphedema: Avoiding the Swollen Arm

Lymphedema describes the swelling that can occur anywhere in the body where the lymphatic system is not draining lymph fluid adequately. Lymph is the clear fluid that bathes the cells of the body and transports waste products of metabolism. When lymphedema occurs in a limb, it is because the fluid cannot drain out of the limb. There are two types of lymphedema: primary and secondary. *Primary lymphedema* occurs because the lymphatic system did not develop correctly in the first place. There are not enough tubes to carry the volume of fluid that accumulates. *Secondary lymphedema* is caused by some form of trauma to the lymphatic system, and most often develops in an arm or leg after lymph node surgery under the arm or in the groin area.

Lymphedema is actually a symptom, not a disease. As related to breast cancer surgery, it is a swelling confined to the arm that results from surgical or radiation treatments. It does not threaten the general health of the rest of the body. You can help prevent it, and it can be treated.

When a woman has an axillary lymph-node dissection, she becomes susceptible to lymphedema. Unfortunately, the possibility of developing swelling in the arm on the side of the surgery lasts for the rest of her life. It could happen a few weeks or months after the surgery, 20 years later, or not at all. The majority of women never develop swelling in the arm. But you must be cautious, and there are steps you can take to protect yourself.

Four years after having a lumpectomy and radiation for breast cancer, Lois developed lymphedema in her arm. (She could also have developed this problem if she had had a mastectomy.) Lois was 52, tall, and slightly overweight. When her arm began to swell, she went back to her surgeon who felt there was nothing he could do. Fortunately, a friend advised Lois not to give up but to seek out someone who could help her. Another friend from her breast cancer support group referred her to me. When she came in for a consultation, I reassured her that there was a great deal that could be done about this problem.

First, we took measurements of the circumference of the arm on her operated side at several points between her hand and her shoulder. Lois was right-handed, and this was her right arm. The measurements showed the circumference was about an inch and a half larger than the left arm.

I asked her if she remembered having any cuts or sores on this hand or arm recently, or any signs of infection.

"Not really," she responded. "The swelling just seemed to come on gradually. I remember having some insect bites on my upper arm a few weeks ago, but nothing happened right away."

She frowned as she studied the difference between her two arms.

"Now my blouses aren't fitting." She looked up. "What can I do?"

I knew Lois needed a lot of information. Unfortunately, she had not received that information when she most needed it: right after having the lymph node surgery under her arm four years ago. Many women's anatomy is such that the "tail" of the breast goes into the armpit area. When this is the case, the lymph vessels in the armpit area are subjected to dual treatments, both surgery and radiation. Radiation can cause *fibrosis* (scar tissue), which can seal off even more lymph vessels. These women may therefore be more susceptible to developing lymphedema. Choosing a lumpectomy to save her breast means that a woman may be increasing her chances of developing visible, chronic swelling in her arm.

I brought out a diagram of the female breast and the lymphatic system (see page 8), and showed Lois where her lymph nodes had been removed for microscopic examination.

"To be graphic," I explained, "the tissue in the armpit area is somewhat like the inside of a pumpkin. It is soft and fatty, and the lymph nodes are like the pumpkin seeds. After the surgeon has removed this tissue, it is the pathologist's job to sort through it, find all the lymph nodes, and mount samples of tissue from each node on slides for examination under a microscope. It's too bad there is no way to put the healthy nodes back.

"The lymph nodes are part of the body's immune system and act as filters. They screen out foreign objects such as bacteria and cancer cells. It's as though you've had the tonsils taken out of your armpit. When the nodes came out, many of the vessels were also unavoidably damaged. Now there aren't as many vessels open to carry fluid.

"Think of the freeway at rush hour, and you close down one lane. There is just as much traffic but not as many lanes to handle it. So you develop a traffic jam. The fluid backs up into the tissue and stagnates. The longer it stays there, the more likely it is to thicken and become hard. The fluid is rich in protein, which invites bacteria to thrive. If the skin is broken and bacteria get in, you can develop an infection rapidly. Your body interprets infection as a fire, and pours more fluid into the arm to put the fire out. The fluid can't get out as fast as it is coming in. This pattern becomes a vicious cycle: infection and edema reinforcing each other. You treat infection by taking an antibiotic. That's the easy part. But then you still have the swelling to deal with. A swollen arm can also easily become reinfected. First we'll talk about skin care and preventive measures; then we'll talk about how to treat the swelling."

I gave Lois a handout on skin-care precautions, a list of protective measures similar to those taught to diabetic patients. First, avoid sharp objects that can break the skin. If you like to work in the garden, wear leather gloves to protect yourself from thorny plants. If you have a cat, be careful not to let it scratch you. Protect yourself from hot objects and biting insects. Do not receive injections in this arm, and do not have blood drawn from this arm. Even though laboratories use sterile needles, it is wise to permanently avoid any type of puncture in this arm. Be sure that clothing and jewelry are not too tight so that marks or indentations are left in your skin. Wash your hands frequently.

Lois and I then reviewed the warning signs of infection in the arm, which is called *cellulitis*. The arm will feel warm to the touch. The skin may change color, becoming red, mottled, or having the appearance of a rash. The arm will probably swell and feel uncomfortable, and the skin might feel itchy. If Lois were to become aware of any or all of these symptoms, she should contact one of her physicians immediately and begin taking an antibiotic. Because these symptoms can come on rapidly, I suggested that Lois carry a prescription for an antibiotic with her when she travels. This would save her the frustration and inconvenience of having to deal with unfamiliar physicians in strange places.

Skin-Care Precautions Following Axillary Lymph-Node Dissection Surgery

1. Wear leather gloves when working in the garden or around thorny plants.

2. Avoid cat scratches.

3. Protect yourself from insect bites: Use repellent or wear long sleeves when around biting insects.

4. Use caution to avoid burns when you are around sources of heat such as the oven or boiling water. If you are burned, immediately apply ice or cold water. Keep the area cold until the burning sensation stops. If a blister forms, cover it with a bandage so that it does not break open.
   Avoid sunburn on this arm.

5. Wear rubber gloves when cleaning with strong detergents, as they can irritate the skin.

6. Use caution when using knives or sharp tools; use a thimble when sewing by hand.

7. Use an electric razor (rather than a blade) when shaving under the arm. Don't try to shave for the first few weeks after the lymph-node surgery.

8. Take good care of your finger nails and cuticles. Keep cuticles soft with cream or lotion so they don't split. Trim hangnails before the skin tears.

9. Avoid wearing clothing or jewelry that is too tight anywhere on this arm. It is important for circulation to be unobstructed.

10. Do not have your blood pressure taken on this arm.

11. Never have injections in this arm. If you have had lymph-node dissections under both arms, have injections in the hip.

12. Do not have blood drawn from this arm. If you have had lymph-node surgery under both arms, have blood drawn from your ankle.

13. Reduce or eliminate salt from your diet. Salt causes fluid to be retained in the tissue.

14. Keep your weight down. Fat acts like a sponge and holds fluid in the arm.

15. Clean any small wound with soap and water. Apply hydrogen peroxide as an antiseptic. Trim away any dead skin that would hold dirt in the wound or block air from getting into the tissue. Bacteria thrive in an environment free of oxygen. Therefore the wound needs to "breathe" to prevent infection. Cover the wound with a thin layer of antibacterial ointment and a bandage. Change the bandage whenever it gets wet or dirty.

16. Be alert for any of the following signs of infection in the arm: a red rash or blotchy area on the skin; skin that feels warm to the touch; swelling, marked tenderness, or persistent itching of the skin. Check your temperature to see if you are developing a fever. All of these symptoms can come on rapidly. Contact your doctor *right away*. You may need to be taking an antibiotic.

It is essential that you practice these skin-care precautions for the operated hand and arm for the rest of your life, *whether or not* you have swelling.

Next we went over basic wound care. I reassured her that everyone gets cuts, scratches, and punctures sooner or later. Clean the wound immediately with mild soap and water. Then use hydrogen peroxide as a local antiseptic. Cover the sore with a thin layer of topical antiseptic ointment and a bandage. Keep it clean and dry until it heals.

There were other steps Lois could take to help herself. She was moderately overweight, so I encouraged her to take off a few pounds. Fat acts like a sponge and holds fluid. Losing even ten pounds can make a significant difference in a chronically swollen arm. It is also important for her to avoid salt in her diet, because salt causes fluid to stay in the tissue.

"Should I take a diuretic?" she asked.

"I don't think so," I responded. "Diuretics act on the kidneys. Your problem is local, not systemic. It is caused by a 'road block' in the lymphatic system where your arm joins your trunk, not by inadequate function of any internal organ. Once in a while a diuretic does help with short-term use. Why don't you talk to your doctor about that? The first step now is to reduce the swelling. If you want to do this the best and most efficient way, I think you should go to a clinic that specializes in lymphedema treatment. We're fortunate because there is one in a city close by."

I gave Lois the address and phone number, and encouraged her to get an appointment right away so that she could hear the treatment options and give herself time to decide what she wanted to do. She understood that she did not have to panic and that there was no rush. The point in moving on this right away was to keep Lois from putting it off and then later regretting that she had lost valuable time. I told Lois that I would assist her as needed.

• • • New Developments in Lymphedema Treatment

The recognition and treatment of lymphedema has changed significantly in the last decade. For years, the standard treatment in this country was the use of *pneumatic compression* (pumping machines) to reduce the swelling, and wearing an elastic compression sleeve on the arm to maintain progress. In the last few years, the technology of these machines has changed, and the cost has gone up. In Europe, England, and

Australia, nurses and therapists have been treating lymphedema with bandaging and manual lymph drainage techniques, which are now becoming more widely practiced in the United States and Canada. Practitioners are now being trained and certified by programs that originated in Europe and Australia, and are now offered in the United States and Canada. The combination of all three techniques—pneumatic compression machines, bandaging, and manual lymph drainage—is now believed to be the best approach to effectively reducing lymphedema. Many physical therapists have lymphedema treatment clinics around the country. The National Lymphedema Network (NLN) can help you locate a clinic near you (see the Resources section at the end of the book).

The NLN is a nonprofit organization established in 1988, based in San Francisco, which delivers information to the public, sponsors conferences and seminars for health professionals, and helps set up new treatment clinics around the country. According to the NLN, there is a small pilot study underway designed to gather preliminary data on a new compression system named the Reid sleeve. Early impressions are that this adjustable sleeve-like device shows promising results for significant reductions in arm swelling. The trend in lymphedema treatment seems to be moving back toward bandaging and compression garments and away from the compression pumps.

Lois went to the clinic and learned about the program. She was offered all three treatments: manual lymph drainage, bandaging the arm with layers of soft padding and low-stretch rolled bandages, and pumping with a sequential gradient pneumatic compression machine. *Manual lymph drainage* (MLD) is a technique of gentle skin stroking and massage designed to open up the lymphatic system in the arm and in the trunk to help the backed-up fluid move out of the arm. Lois could be taught to do the bandaging herself, or, better yet, her partner or a friend could learn how to do it. The pneumatic pumping and MLD were performed at the clinic. Lois could choose to do all or one of the treatments, and she could set up the fre-

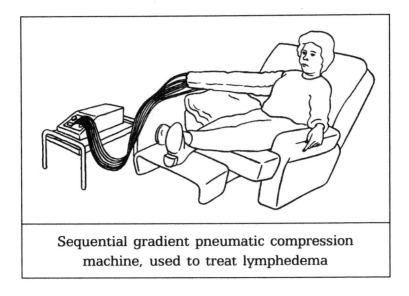

Sequential gradient pneumatic compression machine, used to treat lymphedema

quency of clinic visits based on her schedule and the financial commitment she was willing to make. The more concentrated the program, the faster the results would be.

Lois elected to go for all three treatments: MLD, pumping, and bandaging. She went to the clinic for the pumping and MLD every other day. She took a friend along to learn how to help her with the bandaging at home. The bandaging involves three layers. First, a special gauze is wrapped around individual fingers and is continued up the arm. A second layer of padding is then added for compression. The third layer is a low-stretch bandage. Each layer begins at the fingers and progresses up the arm, toward the heart.

For the first week, Lois wore the bandages day and night except when she showered. Lois called to ask about exercising her arm. I told her that it was very important to move her arm as normally as possible when the bandages are on. The action of the muscles pumping against the firm resistance of the bandage helps to move the fluid up and out of the arm. It is also good to open and close the fingers, bend and straighten the elbow, raise and lower the arm, and perform other usual activities. Lois had to avoid lifting heavy objects or doing vigorous

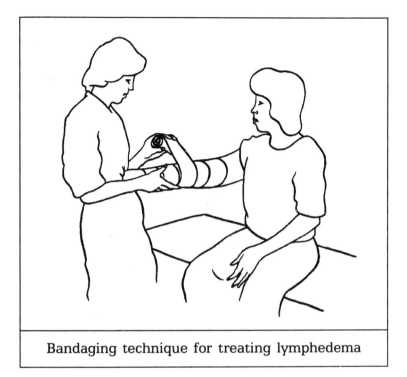

Bandaging technique for treating lymphedema

repetitive motions against a resistance, such as rubbing, scrubbing, pushing, or pulling with this arm.

An important issue for Lois was handling the cosmetic impact of the bandages. Of course they were very visible and she knew they would draw unwanted attention. We talked about this for some time. I pointed out that the bandages were temporary, and that the future health of her arm was more important than what other people thought. We practiced coming up with things to say when people asked her what happened to her arm, and we shared a good laugh over the one liners we came up with. Lois' favorite was: "You should see the other guy!"

After about two weeks, the measurements of the circumference of Lois' arm leveled off, indicating that the treatments had accomplished a major reduction. Lois was then ready to be fitted with an elastic compression sleeve to maintain her progress. The swelling had come down to the point that her right

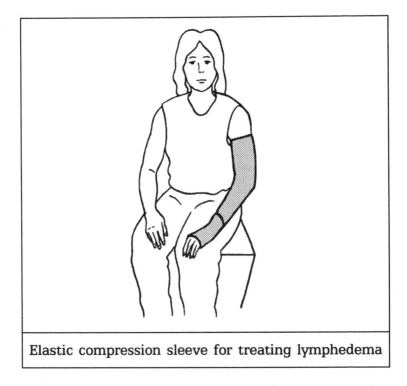

Elastic compression sleeve for treating lymphedema

arm was only a half inch larger than the left arm. Compared to the bandages, the sleeve was easy to put on and a lot more comfortable to wear. She wore the sleeve faithfully for several months, then gradually began to reduce the time she wore it.

She lost fifteen pounds by changing her eating habits and committing herself to daily exercise. Losing this weight and keeping it off would help prevent further swelling. She read up on how to reduce the amount of fat in her diet and changed the way she was preparing food. She learned that just walking briskly or cycling for 20 to 30 minutes every day, fast enough to bring her heart rate up to an exercise level, proved to be very effective aerobic exercise. She arranged to walk with a friend, which she knew would help keep her motivated.

Six months later, Lois came back to report on her progress. She smiled as she shared her accomplishments with me and there was an unmistakable look of pride on her face. She asked again about exercising the arm.

"Continue to avoid repetitive motions against a resistance," I advised. "Too much pushing, pulling, rubbing, scrubbing, lifting, or carrying heavy objects can cause the swelling to come back again. This is because the muscles in your arm need fluid to feed them when they are working hard. Then more fluid goes into the arm than can get out. It takes some trial and error to learn the difference between use and abuse.

"I want to be sure you understand that it is *also* very important to exercise this arm in a healthy way. This means *do* keep your muscles strong and your joints mobile. Don't avoid using this arm for your usual daily activities. Normal movements keep the muscles active, which keeps the fluid moving. You already have excellent mobility. We need to be sure that you keep good muscle tone to stimulate good circulation. If you see the swelling coming back, wear your compression sleeve when you do any activity that requires continuous hand or arm movements. Your arm muscles working against the pressure of the garment keeps the fluid moving. Whenever you travel in higher elevations or on an airplane, wear your sleeve; the change in atmospheric pressure can also bring the swelling back."

All of this information made good sense to Lois. As she prepared to leave, she told me: "This was a hard experience to go through. I thought all of the trauma of breast cancer was behind me. Then this new problem came up. It helped me realize that taking care of myself is an ongoing responsibility. Just because I'm well now doesn't mean I should take my health for granted again."

••• What Do I Say to My Daughter? Breast Self-Examination and Preventive Measures

Many women who survive breast cancer worry about how to help their teenage and adult daughters protect themselves. They want to help their daughters be aware and careful without frightening them. The first step is to find the best way to share your own personal experience with your daughter. This means being open with your fears and frustrations, yet keeping everything in perspective.

An important preventive measure to pass on to your daughter is breast self-examination (BSE). Every young woman needs to learn this procedure, particularly those who have a close relative who has had the disease. Mammograms are not dependable as a diagnostic tool for younger women (those in their twenties and thirties) because their breast tissue is too dense and fibrous to allow a clear picture. There is no doubt that mammograms are very effective in diagnosing tumors in women 50 and older, but there is still debate about the ideal frequency and timing of mammograms for women between 40 and 50. The majority of lumps are still discovered by the women themselves.

Every woman, whether or not she has had breast surgery and no matter what her age, should become familiar with how her breasts feel to the touch. The earlier a woman starts this practice, the more effective it is. Sometime in her twenties, a woman needs to learn the technique and establish a routine of self-examination each month a few days after her period is over, when her breasts are least dense and the easiest to feel. After menopause, she can choose one day of the month, perhaps the date of her birthday.

Probably the best person to teach a young woman how to do self-examination and to be comfortable with it is a female doctor, nurse, or nurse practitioner who is trained to do this. There are many breast diagnostic clinics and mammography centers that have specially trained staff members. The American Cancer Society also has self-instruction brochures, and can refer women to these centers as well as to appropriate health care practitioners.

Some women who have had breast cancer mean well and intend to protect their daughters by keeping information about their diagnosis and treatment from them. However, this approach often causes more fear in the long run than it prevents. Once again, communication is the key. Most women who have been through this experience believe that information

Breast Self-Examination

1. Stand in front of a mirror. Look at your breasts carefully in the following four positions: arms at your sides, reaching up overhead, pressing your hands on your hips, and bending forward.

   Look for changes in the shape and contour of your breasts, or changes in the skin texture such as puckering or dimpling.

   Then squeeze each nipple and look for any discharge.

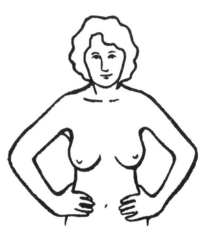

2. Lie on your back with a folded towel or pillow under your left shoulder. Use the flat surface of three fingers of your right hand to feel your left breast. Press down and make slow, circular motions.

   Start at the outer edge of the breast and work in toward the nipple. You can examine your breasts in circles, strips, or quadrants. Cover the entire breast and the underarm area. You are looking for any lump that feels harder than the rest of the breast tissue.

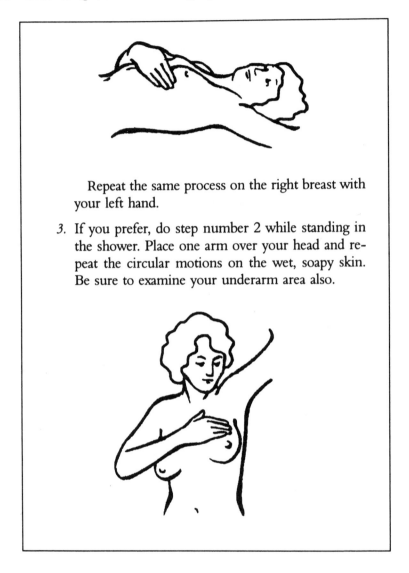

Repeat the same process on the right breast with your left hand.

3. If you prefer, do step number 2 while standing in the shower. Place one arm over your head and repeat the circular motions on the wet, soapy skin. Be sure to examine your underarm area also.

delivered clearly and gently at the right time for their daughter to absorb is the best approach. Teenagers and even pre-teens report that they were actually relieved when their mother showed them her mastectomy scar, radiation site, or reconstructed breast. The unknown always seems to be more anxiety-producing than the known.

Women who have a strong family history of breast cancer need to take extra precautions. A strong family history means that more than one woman in their immediate family (grandmother, mother, aunt, sister, or even daughter) has had the disease. These women should have a baseline mammogram when they are in their thirties, or even earlier if the family tendency is to develop the disease early. Some seriously consider having prophylactic mastectomies before they develop disease. By choosing to have their breasts removed as a prevention (with or without reconstruction, depending on the woman), they are able to save their lymphatic system, because axillary lymph-node dissection surgery is not necessary if cancer is not detected. For any woman who feels that her family history makes her a walking time bomb, choosing to take aggressive action early saves her body from unnecessary complications, as well as bringing her—and others around her—peace of mind.

Young women can also protect themselves by developing good health habits early. Although the causes of breast cancer are not yet known, the research and theories are plentiful. It is certainly safe to say it is wise to be aware of what we put into our bodies. Anything women can do to influence their daughters not to smoke, to limit the amount of fat in their diets, to eat lots of fresh vegetables, fruit, and fiber, and to exercise regularly, is energy well spent. As more cancer-causing chemicals become identified, young women should avoid them when possible. And of course, the behavior you want to encourage is best promoted by setting a good example in your own life. How you choose to live your life after experiencing breast cancer can be the most powerful influence of all.

••• Protecting Yourself from the Fear of Recurrence

All women who have once experienced breast cancer fear that it might return. This is a very normal fear, and you can help protect yourself from a recurrence. First, schedule and keep your appointments for follow-up examinations with your doctors. For some time after your treatments are complete, you will need to see your surgeon, your oncologist, or your family physician every few months. I tell my patients to think of these physicians as your invaluable committee of consultants. You pay them to do the worrying for you. *Always* report any unusual symptom such as a new lump or pain unrelated to direct trauma *right away.* Don't wait for a scheduled appointment. Don't think you are being silly or worry that you are wasting your doctor's time. Your doctors are hired consultants, and they are there to help keep you well. It is your responsibility to utilize their skill.

Everyone finds pain the most deceptive symptom to analyze and report. Many women worry too much about every innocent discomfort they experience, often forgetting that this same sensation used to occur long before they had cancer. Others may diminish the importance of a serious signal from their body. Guidelines about how to interpret and report pain are on page 93.

Five years after having a lumpectomy, axillary lymph-node dissection and radiation, Maria had recurring episodes of shoulder and upper-arm pain that worried her. Maria was a tall, energetic woman of 54. She went to her doctor, who diagnosed tendinitis and referred her to a physical therapist. She was quite relieved to learn that she had a common ailment. As we worked with her shoulder, she asked a question I had heard many times before.

"I panic easily when I develop a new pain," she said. "How do I know when not to worry?"

I told Maria that this was a normal reaction. "Having cancer robs you of your sense of safety. Cancer survivors worry that any new symptom in their body means that the cancer has come back. There are, however, some guidelines to go by to reduce unnecessary anxiety. Pain always has a pattern. It is important to look for that pattern. Is the pain worse during the day when you are active, and then better after rest? Is it worse at night and then relieved by activity during the day? Fortu-

How to Describe Pain to Your Doctor

1. How Does the Pain Feel?
   Aching
   Sore
   Sharp
   Throbbing

2. How Strong Is the Pain?
   Assign the pain a number value on a scale of one to ten, with ten as very bad. For example: it may be a three when you are lying down, and a seven when you stand up; it may be a four at bedtime and a two when you wake up in the morning.

3. Where Is the Pain?
   Locate the place in your body as clearly as you can. Does it move around or is it always in the same place?

4. When Does the Pain Occur?
   When you are resting? When you are active?
   When you are standing, sitting, lying down, walking, or moving a part of your body?
   Daytime, nighttime, or both?
   Before eating, or after eating?

5. What Intensifies It? What Relieves It?
   Moving the part?
   Sitting down? Lying down?
   Standing up? Walking?
   Heat? Cold?

nately, most pain that is caused by inflammation of or trauma to soft tissue is quite predictable. This type of pain can usually be influenced by movement or position. If you can make the pain better or worse by moving the limb, reaching, lifting, standing up, sitting down, or lying down, it is probably caused by a common problem unrelated to cancer. Even pain from pinched nerves in the neck or back, which often radiates down the arm or leg, tends to follow this pattern.

"One of the most common sources of pain is muscle tension caused by static posture or internalized stress. Overworked and fatigued muscles express themselves with aching and cramping pain, often in the neck, shoulder-blade area, or lower back. Muscle tension headaches are set off by continuous spasms of the neck muscles, and usually radiate up over the scalp and into the forehead and eyes."

Maria laughed out loud. "Will you make me a 'worry chart' so I can keep track of the good pain and the bad pain?"

I thought about it and decided that wasn't such a bad idea. I suggested that she write down the times and activities that intensified or relieved her pain. Then she could make a graph and see the pattern clearly for herself. Worry seems to amplify pain. The better you understand your pain and are able to describe it to someone, the less it will frighten you. It is usually easier to cope with pain than with fear.

EIGHT

Emotional Issues

For more than 25 years, women have been sharing their stories of pain and courage with me. Repeatedly, they have urged me to write about their experiences of recovering. They have taught me what their physical and emotional needs are, and they have taught me about their deepest fears. The following sections touch on these insights.

Our bodies talk to us all the time. They have a language all their own. Illness forces us to listen to them and take action. A health crisis also intensifies the relationships we have with the important people in our lives. Breast cancer survivors seem to have an inside track on these issues, and they tend to be very outspoken about what they have learned. Many of their feelings are expressed here.

· · · Messages from Your Body

Helen was a petite, soft-spoken woman in her early fifties. As we worked together to restore her shoulder motion, she shared some very personal feelings.

"Sometimes I think I brought this on myself," she said.

"What do you mean?"

"This has been a terribly stressful year for me. My mother died earlier this year. She had been ill for a long time, and I had her move in with my husband and me. Caring for her and working full time was very exhausting. That she was living with us proved to be very hard on my relationship with my husband. I think he really resented her being there. He withdrew by becoming a workaholic and spending long hours at the office. I feel guilty because I can't take care of everybody's needs, even though I know that it's ridiculous to have that expectation. I've felt so inadequate. Maybe I made myself sick."

This was not the first time I had heard this. The response I gave Helen represented what I have heard throughout my career: the thoughtful experiences of so many women who have been through this same health crisis.

"I'm a messenger," I told her. "And I will pass on to you what I have learned from other patients. It takes a lot of courage to cope with learning that you have a life-threatening disease. By courage, I mean the willingness to face your own worst fears and still move forward. There are many unknowns. You have to make difficult decisions and hope you did your homework well enough.

"In our culture, many women find it difficult to adequately take care of their own needs. They put their energy and time into their husbands, children, parents, career, and community projects. They easily forget about themselves. When I ask my patients to make a list of their most important priorities before their illness, they often do not even list their own personal needs or pleasures.

"I firmly believe that illness is one of nature's finest teachers. Having a health crisis forces you to reorganize your priorities. Learning that you have cancer puts a very different perspective on events and relationships. Many women find the courage to make important decisions that may change their lives forever. Some discover that they are now strong enough to get out of unhealthy relationships. Others are able to strengthen relationships that are basically good ones, because these terrifying events draw them closer to the important people in their lives.

"Some women make career changes or stop working altogether. They may recognize that a stressful job is no longer worth the psychological toll it takes. Some women take on a project they may have always wanted to do, even if it is unpopular or not financially secure. It may become very important to do something that has been an unfulfilled dream, because it can no longer be put off."

Helen was taking all this in intently. I located a notepad and sat down beside her, then drew a diagram to illustrate my next point.

"Let's suppose that disease has three components." I drew a circle and divided it into three sections. "Here is the section called genetic predisposition. These are the genes you inher-

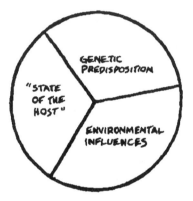

ited from your mother and father. They may or may not influence the likelihood of your developing breast cancer. Unfortunately, you don't get to vote in this category. The next section we'll label environmental influences: the air we breathe, the food we eat, the chemicals we are exposed to every day that may cause cancer. Perhaps we get to vote on half of these issues. Sometimes we can choose not to be exposed to agents that we know may be harmful. The third slice of the pie is the area where you do get to vote on everything. We shall call this portion the 'state of the host.' That means your body's disease-fighting mechanisms. How healthy is your immune system? How can you influence your own ability to be well? Remember, it takes years for a breast tumor to become large enough to feel or even be seen on a mammogram.

"There are several issues to be considered in this third section of the pie. There is no question about the importance of good nutrition. All you have to do is pick up a newspaper to read the latest ideas about a healthy diet. Most people in our culture do not eat enough fruits and vegetables. Scientists are confirming what our grandmothers have told us for generations: foods such as broccoli, garlic, and soybeans are good for us. Not only that, they are learning that many fruits and vegetables have cancer-fighting properties. Regular exercise is another important consideration. My suggestion is to keep it simple. Commit yourself to one half-hour of brisk walking, cycling, or swimming every day or every other day. You don't need to put yourself through intense physical training or be a competitive athlete. Just give your heart, lungs, and muscles a good, regular workout.

"Now let's examine ways in which stress can influence this 'state of the host.'

"Here is a different way to look at the stress in your life." I drew a second diagram. "Think of your body as a pressure cooker. You bolt down the lid and turn up the fire. Let's focus on what is boiling inside the pot creating all the pressure. The ingredients of your emotional stew are some old familiar feelings: fear, anger, guilt, and resentment. Even though these emotions can be very negative, they are not the real problem. The fact that we tend to hold these feelings in and 'sit on them' is what causes the pressure to build. We don't acknowledge to ourselves or to other people concerned that we have these feelings. We don't express them appropriately or at the right time. It's not the problem that is the problem, it's the *denial* of the problem that is the problem!

"The steam valve keeps the lid from blowing off the pressure cooker. Your body looks for its own steam valve to release its pressure. Your body recognizes the suppressed emotion even if you don't, and will find some way to release it. When some people are anxious or resentful, they may develop headaches, an upset stomach, skin rashes, or a variety of other common stress-related ailments. These ailments are the 'steam

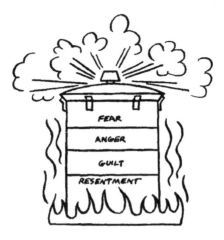

valves' that release internal pressure as physical symptoms. What's important is that when your body speaks to you, be sure you are listening. Once you recognize and acknowledge the emotion underlying the symptom, you have the power to reverse it. Perhaps this philosophy can apply to major disease as well. There is certainly a demonstrated connection between stress and heart attacks."

Helen's eyes widened with insight. She looked at the diagram of the pressure cooker and put her finger right on the word "anger."

"That's my problem area. I've been very angry for a long time, but I'm afraid to express it. I guess I learned not to show anger from my mother. I think she never felt she was able to take charge of her life. She turned her anger in on herself. Unfortunately, she was not a good model for me. I have a tendency to punish myself when I don't take charge of my feelings."

"Congratulations!" I smiled at her. "You've made an important discovery. Find someone you trust with whom you can talk about this. If you don't have a close friend you feel comfortable with, consider a professional."

There are many excellent licensed marriage and family counselors, social workers, clinical psychologists, and breast cancer support groups available as resources. Local mental health facilities, physicians, and the American Cancer Society can refer you to the appropriate professionals for individual or group counseling. There are breast cancer support groups at many hospitals and large outpatient clinics. Staff members in your hospital's mental health or social services department have information about support groups. These groups are usually free to participants or require a nominal charge. See the Resources, pages 107–108, for regional and national support organizations.

Helen pursued help in both breast cancer support groups and professional counseling. I kept in touch with her for a long time and watched her make some remarkable changes in her life. Years later, she told me that having cancer had actually proven to be a gift. She would never have made the changes that she now believes actually saved her life, if she had not had to face a life-threatening disease.

• • • Who Is Your Partner

I have observed two rather common patterns of strain that this health crisis places on primary relationships. The first pattern I call the rejection–withdrawal cycle. The woman undergoing treatment may feel as though she is no longer sexually attractive to her partner. After breast surgery, she may imagine his repulsion or anticipate his rejection and withdraw from him. Her partner reacts to this withdrawal and interprets it as rejection of him. He in turn withdraws from her. They can become locked in a vicious cycle of withdrawal and rejection. However, touching and talking to each other can break this cycle. Sometimes they need the help of a concerned third person to intervene and facilitate communication. It often only requires a frank conversation to expose the myths that are perpetuating the misunderstanding and unhappiness. The woman is often startled to hear her partner say that he is terrified that he will lose her. What is happening to her breast is not his main concern at all. He may also

be fearful of physically hurting her during lovemaking because she has had surgery in such a sensitive area. An added
problem may be that their timing is off: when one of them is
focused on immediate concerns, the other is thinking about
the future. If at this point her partner is able to reassure her
that he loves her just the way she is, probably more than
ever, and that her body is not more important to him than
she is, the problem can be resolved.

When Rebecca and I were working on her shoulder exercises, she talked a great deal about her partner, Dan. She was
worried about how he was handling everything that was happening to her. It seemed to her that he was afraid to talk about
any of his feelings. I suggested that she bring him in for a
treatment session. I hoped that if we could get him directly
involved in Rebecca's recovery, it could give him the opportunity to open himself up to her. When they learned the partner
exercise (page 60), I could see that something important was
happening to them.

During the following session with Rebecca, she told me that
someone else giving Dan permission to touch her had proven
to be the icebreaker. Somehow, participating in a structured
activity where Dan was touching Rebecca helped him over-
come his feelings of isolation. Now they were both talking
about their feelings, and Rebecca was thrilled that they had
been able to make this breakthrough.

The second relationship pattern is more complex. This occurs when the woman's husband or partner is not willing or
able to emotionally handle the crisis. When I asked Margot to
bring along her husband, Jack, to assist with the isometric exercises, I sensed right away that there was a problem. She was
sure he would not come. After we talked about it for a while,
she realized that she did not even want him to come. She
knew that their relationship was failing, and now she could no
longer ignore that fact. Her diagnosis with cancer had become
a wake-up call for the future of her marriage.

Unfortunately for Margot, she needed support and assis-
tance right now. As I have seen happen many times, Margot

found that support in several of her women friends. All she had to do was ask. One friend drove her to her treatment sessions. Another came and learned the isometric exercise program. A third took over the home front, arranging for meals to be prepared for Margot and her two teenage children. Margot confided with me later that these three friends had been deeply affected by the whole experience. Their opportunity to participate had been just as meaningful to them as it had been to her.

Two years after completing her treatments, Margot came to see me for an unrelated injury requiring therapy and she filled me in on her life. She had gone through a difficult and painful divorce. She reported that now her life was going in a completely new and positive direction. I was impressed by how vibrant she looked. She offered some valuable insights about the impact that facing a life-threatening disease can have on a primary relationship. She suggested that women in this situation ask themselves some important questions. First: who in your life is willing and able to help you with these feelings? Second: is that person truly there for you, wanting to give you the necessary time and support? Third: if there are unresolved differences between you, are you both able to put them on hold during this crisis? Fourth and probably most important: is this the person you want to be with you throughout this critical experience, when the chips are really down?

••• What Makes a Survivor?

Whenever I have the opportunity to visit with the women who have kept in touch with me over the years, they talk about the attitudes and behaviors they believe help them to be survivors. What do these woman have in common, and what do they do? My observation is that they practice an attitude of determination to live well. This usually means that they have made some permanent changes in their lifestyles. They have learned how to take better care of themselves, physically and psychologically. They have developed a better understanding of their own needs and limitations.

One quality they say is important is self-confidence. They describe this in different ways: some emphasize being more assertive; others talk about being less fearful and using more common sense. They all are aware of how much more precious time is to them. Many of these women feel that they may have spent their lives trying to please others. Now they take the time and effort to figure out what they want for themselves, and how to get it. When facing a new challenge, they ask themselves: "Does this make me feel good about me?" They say they are learning the differences between being selfless, selfish, and self-aware.

One woman quoted from a book she was reading: "Ships are safe in the harbor, but that's not what ships are designed for." She told me she is now much more willing to take risks than she was before her illness.

Another said, "It isn't so much whether I get sick again, as how I live in the meantime. I used to feel guilty about everything that didn't go right. Now, I'm not going to waste my energy flagellating myself and wonder why I didn't do things differently."

I have observed that these survivors also have a good sense of humor. Most important, they know how to laugh at themselves. They seem to have learned that they can bring about their own happiness. They tell me that it takes courage to be happy. They do not waste their energy blaming themselves or other people or events for their illness.

A crucial element these women describe is the role of the important people who are now in their lives. Many describe unwavering support from the people who love them and believe in them. This is not the same as having constant attention. On the contrary, many of these survivors have spent a great deal of time alone. Some are very happy being single; others are single parents. The point here is that these survivors have become more selective in their primary relationships: they have learned to surround themselves with people who value them. They work hard to honor and nourish their friendships. They are no longer willing to tolerate emotional abuse or neglect.

To me, these women are stronger because of their experiences with breast cancer. They go on with their lives with new insights that they learned the hard way. They have a different perspective on life because they have faced a life-threatening disease. They seem to value themselves more than they did before their illness. And they want to help each other.

Many of them become volunteers in organizations that offer support, distribute information, and promote funding for breast-cancer research. Others participate in support groups. Some write about their experiences. And all of them are changed by having had this disease.

Recommended Reading

Bailey, Covert, and Bishop, Lea, *The Fit or Fat Woman* (Boston: Houghton Mifflin Company, 1989).

Bailey, Covert, *The New Fit or Fat* (Boston: Houghton Mifflin Company, 1991).
Both of Covert Bailey's books are excellent resources for anyone who is interested in fitness and aerobic exercise. I believe his expertise in this area is unsurpassed.

Benedet, Rosalind, N.P., MSN, *Healing: A Woman's Guide to Recovery After Mastectomy* (San Francisco: R. Benedet Publishing, 1993).
Practical information for coping with the emotional and physical aftermath of mastectomy.

Bruning, Nancy, *Breast Implants: Everything You Need to Know* (Alameda CA: Hunter House, 1995).
A thorough report on breast implants, including the surgical procedures, the different products available, and their risks and benefits.

Davidson, James, M.D., and Winebrenner, Jan, *In Touch with Your Breasts* (Waco TX: WRS Publishing, 1995).
A digest of questions and answers covering all aspects of breast care.

Kradjian, Robert M., M.D., *Save Yourself from Breast Cancer* (New York: Berkley Books, 1994).
A compelling scientific presentation advocating diet and exercise to prevent breast cancer, written by a breast surgeon.

LaTour, Kathy, *The Breast Cancer Companion* (New York: Avon Books, 1993).
This is an excellent overall resource covering medical, physical, and emotional issues, written by a breast cancer survivor.

Love, Susan M., M.D., *Dr. Susan Love's Breast Book* (Reading MA: Addison-Wesley Publishing, 1990).
Dr. Love's book has become the "working Bible" of breast cancer resources, written by a prominent breast surgeon.

McGinn, Kerry A., R.N., *The Informed Woman's Guide to Breast Health* (Palo Alto CA: Bull Publishing, 1992).
An excellent resource on breast symptoms and changes that are not cancerous.

McGinn, Kerry A., R.N., and Haylock, Pamela J., R.N., *Women's Cancers* (Alameda CA: Hunter House, 1993).
A complete guide to approaching the diagnosis, treatment, and emotional issues surrounding breast and gynecologic cancers, written by two oncology nurses. It includes a detailed section on breast cancer.

Sicard-Rosenbaum, et al., "Effects of Continuous Therapeutic Ultrasound on Growth and Metastasis of Subcutaneous Murine Tumors," *Physical Therapy* Vol 75 No. 1, January 1995.
A recent scientific study on the effects of ultrasound on tumors in laboratory mice.

Get Up and Go After Breast Surgery (an exercise videotape), developed in consultation with the Michigan Chapter of the American Cancer Society and the University of Michigan.
Available through Health Tapes, Inc., 13320 Northend, Oak Park MI 48237, (810) 548-2500.

Resources

American Cancer Society (national headquarters)
1599 Clifton Road, N. E.
Atlanta GA 30329
(404) 329-7623
Contact ACS national headquarters for the location of your local chapter for information on free services and literature for cancer patients and their families.

American Physical Therapy Association
1111 N. Fairfax Street
Alexandria VA 22314-1488
(703) 684-2782
The APTA can help you find local physical therapists with an interest in cancer patients.

Breast Cancer Physical Therapy Center
1905 Spruce Street
Philadelphia PA 19103
(215) 772-0160
Linda Miller, P.T.
The Center can refer you to physical therapists who specialize in lymphedema treatment and who are practicing in clinics in various locations around the United States.

The Community Breast Health Project
770 Welch Road, Suite 370
Palo Alto CA 94304
(415) 494-1856

The Project provides information about all aspects of breast health care, including treatment, education, and support services. The Project has recently established a computer connection with the Internet, which ties it to cancer resources all over the world.

National Alliance of Breast Cancer Organizations (NABCO)
9 East 37th Street, Tenth Floor
New York NY 10016
(212) 889-0606
National resource for information on all aspects of breast cancer with 300 member organizations.

National Lymphedema Network
2211 Post Street, Suite 404
San Francisco CA 94115-3427
1-800-541-3259
A nonprofit organization that offers information on the prevention and treatment of lymphedema.

Index

LYMPHEDEMA: A Breast Cancer Patient's Guide to Prevention and Healing by Jeannie Burt & Gwen White, P.T.

This book emphasizes active self-help for lymphedema, the disfiguring and often painful swelling, particularly of the arm, that affects as many as 30 percent of breast cancer patients. It describes the many options women have for preventing and treating the condition, ranging from exercise to compression to massage.

"A very useful book for patients...a good practical resource for professionals." — Saskia J. Thiadens, R.N., Ex. Dir., National Lymphedema Network

224 pages ... 50 illus. ... Paperback $12.95 ... Hardcover $22.95

WOMEN'S CANCERS: How to Prevent Them, How to Treat Them, How to Beat Them
by Kerry A. McGinn, R.N. and Pamela J. Haylock, R.N.

Women's Cancers is the first book to focus specifically on the cancers that affect only women—breast, cervical, ovarian, and uterine. It offers the latest information in a clear style and discusses all the issues, from the psychological to the practical, surrounding a cancer diagnosis.

"WOMEN'S CANCERS is fully comprehensive, helpful to patients and healthcare workers alike. Recommended." — LIBRARY JOURNAL

512 pages ... 68 illus. ... 2nd ed. ... Paperback $19.95 ... Hardcover $29.95

THE FEISTY WOMAN'S BREAST CANCER BOOK
by Elaine Ratner

This personal, advice-packed guide helps women navigate the emotional and psychological landscape surrounding breast cancer, and make their own decisions with confidence. Its insight and positive message make this a perfect companion for every feisty woman who wants not only to survive but thrive after breast cancer.

"There are times when a woman needs a wise and level-headed friend, someone kind, savvy and, and caring...[This] book...is just such a friend..." —Rachel Naomi Remen, M.D., author of *Kitchen Table Wisdom*

288 pages ... Paperback $14.95 ... Hardcover $24.95

To order books see last page or call (800) 266-5592

CANCER—INCREASING YOUR ODDS FOR SURVIVAL: A Resource Guide for Integrating Mainstream, Alternative and Complementary Therapies

by David Bognar

Based on the four-part television series hosted by Walter Cronkite, this book provides a comprehensive look at traditional medical treatments for cancer and how these can be supplemented. It explains the basics of cancer and the best actions to take immediately after a diagnosis of cancer. It outlines the various conventional, alternative, and complementary treatments; describes the powerful effect the mind can have on the body and the therapies that strengthen this connection; and explores spiritual healing and issues surrounding death and dying. Includes full-length interviews with leaders in the field of healing, including Joan Borysenko, Stephen Levine, and Bernie Siegel.

352 pages ... Paperback $15.95 ... Hard cover $25.95

CANCER DOESN'T HAVE TO HURT: How to Conquer the Pain Caused by Cancer and Cancer Treatment

by Pamela J. Haylock, R.N., and Carol P. Curtiss, R.N.

Studies have shown that people with cancer benefit by taking control over the treatment of the disease and of their pain. Written with warmth and clarity by two oncology nurses with more than 50 years of experience between them, this guide explains cancer pain, explores the emotional effects on sufferers and caregivers, and shows readers how to manage pain using a combination of medical and natural self-help treatments. Includes a "Self-Care Workbook" section.

192 pages ... 10 illus. ... Paperback $14.95 ... Hard cover $24.95

HOW WOMEN CAN *FINALLY* STOP SMOKING

by Robert C. Klesges, Ph.D., and Margaret DeBon

Strategies for quitting are different for men and women. Women who quit smoking tend to gain more weight, menstrual cycles and menopause affect the likelihood of success, and their withdrawal symptoms are different. This program is based on the highly successful model at Memphis State University and is authored by pioneers in the field.

192 pages ... 3 illus. ... Paperback ... $11.95

To order books see last page or call (800) 266-5592

MENOPAUSE WITHOUT MEDICINE *Revised 3rd Edition*
by Linda Ojeda, Ph.D.

Linda Ojeda broke new ground when she began her study of nonmedical approaches to menopause more than ten years ago. In this update of her classic book, she discusses natural sources of estrogen; how mood swings are affected by diet and personality; and the newest research on osteoporosis, breast cancer, and heart disease. She thoroughly examines the hormone therapy debate; suggests natural remedies for depression, hot flashes, sexual changes, and skin and hair problems. As seen in Time magazine.

352 pages ... 40 illus. ... Paperback $14.95 ... Hardcover $23.95

THE NATURAL ESTROGEN DIET: Healthy Recipes for Perimenopause and Menopause
by Dr. Lana Liew with Linda Ojeda, Ph.D.

Two women's health and nutrition experts offer women almost 100 easy and delicious recipes to naturally increase their level of estrogen. Each recipe includes nutritional information such as the calorie, cholesterol, and calcium content. They also provide an overview of how estrogen can be derived from the food we eat, describe which foods are the highest in estrogen content, and offer meal plan ideas.

224 pages ... 25 illus. ... Paperback $13.95

HER HEALTHY HEART: A Woman's Guide to Preventing and Reversing Heart Disease Naturally
by Linda Ojeda, Ph.D.

Heart disease is the #1 killer of American women ages 44 to 65, yet most of the research is done on men. HER HEALTHY HEART fills this gap by addressing the unique aspects of heart disease in women and natural ways to combat it. Dr. Ojeda explains how women can prevent heart disease whether they take hormone replacement therapy (HRT) or not. She also provides information on how women can reduce their risk of heart disease by making changes in diet, increasing physical activity, and managing stress. A 50-item lifestyle questionnaire helps women discover areas to work on for heath health.

352 pages ... 7 illus. ... Paperback $14.95 ... Hard cover $24.95

To order books see last page or call (800) 266-5592

ORDER FORM

10% DISCOUNT on orders of $50 or more —
20% DISCOUNT on orders of $150 or more —
30% DISCOUNT on orders of $500 or more —
On cost of books for fully prepaid orders

NAME

ADDRESS

CITY/STATE   ZIP/POSTCODE

PHONE   COUNTRY (outside of U.S.)

TITLE	QTY	PRICE	TOTAL
Recovering From Breast Surgery		@ $11.95	
Lymphedema		@ $12.95	

Prices subject to change without notice

Please list other titles below:

		@ $	
		@ $	
		@ $	
		@ $	
		@ $	
		@ $	
		@ $	

Check here to receive our book catalog ☐   FREE

Shipping Costs:
First book: $3.00 by book post ($4.50 by UPS, Priority Mail, or to ship outside the U.S.)
Each additional book: $1.00
For rush orders and bulk shipments call us at (800) 266-5592

TOTAL	
Less discount @_____%	( )
TOTAL COST OF BOOKS	
Calif. residents add sales tax	
Shipping & handling	
TOTAL ENCLOSED	

Please pay in U.S. funds only

☐ Check ☐ Money Order ☐ Visa ☐ Mastercard ☐ Discover

Card #_____ Exp. date_____

Signature_____

Complete and mail to:
Hunter House Inc., Publishers
PO Box 2914, Alameda CA 94501-0914
Orders: (800) 266-5592   email: ordering@hunterhouse.com
Phone (510) 865-5282 Fax (510) 865-4295
☐ Check here to receive our book catalog

RBS-R2 11/99